Marc Abraham grew up in London's leafy suburbia
with his mum, dad, sister and a host of furry creatures.
He spent countless hours in the back garden with his
butterfly net in the faithful company of Suzy the cat and
Speedy the tortoise. Setting his heart on becoming a vet
he went off to train at Edinburgh University. Before
setting up his own emergency practice in Brighton he
worked as a locum, but his career has been peppered
with globe-trotting adventures; from treating racehorses
in Kentucky, rescuing stray dogs and cats in Tsunami-hit
Thailand, to conservation work in the Amazon rain-
forest. Never off duty, he even once delivered a litter of
puppies in a bar in Val D'Isere!

Marc is the resident vet on both ITV's *This Morning*
and BBC's *Breakfast*. He has co-presented Crufts and
Sky1's *My Pet Shame* with *Gavin & Stacey*'s Joanna Page.
He supports a range of animal charities, and campaigns
against animal cruelty such as puppy farming. In 2007 he
was voted 'The UK's Favourite Vet' by the British public.

www.marcthevet.com

1 3 5 7 9 10 8 6 4 2

First published in 2011 by Ebury Press, an imprint of Ebury Publishing
A Random House Group company

Copyright © Marc Abraham 2011

Marc Abraham has asserted his right to be identified as the author of this work
in accordance with the Copyright, Designs and Patents Act 1988

The Random House Group Limited Reg. No. 954009

Addresses for companies within the Random House Group can be found at
www.randomhouse.co.uk

A CIP catalogue record for this book is available from the British Library

The Random House Group Limited supports The Forest Stewardship
Council (FSC), the leading international forest certification organisation.
All our titles that are printed on Greenpeace approved FSC certified paper
carry the FSC logo. Our paper procurement policy can be
found at www.rbooks.co.uk/environment

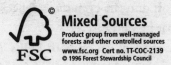

Mixed Sources

Product group from well-managed
forests and other controlled sources
www.fsc.org Cert no. TT-COC-2139
© 1996 Forest Stewardship Council

Designed and set by seagulls.net

Printed in the UK by CPI Cox & Wyman, Reading, RG1 8EX

ISBN 9780091937874

To buy books by your favourite authors and register for offers visit
www.rbooks.co.uk

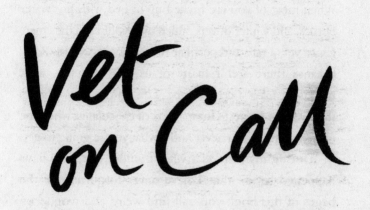

My First Year as an Out-of-Hours Vet

MARC ABRAHAM

Author's Note

When most of you are tucked up in bed with hot water bottles, and winter duvets pulled over your ears, the emergency vet, a rare and peculiar breed, goes to work. Rare, because there aren't many of us, and peculiar, well, because it takes a certain type. Life on the out-of-hours shift was like Forrest Gump's box of chocolates: when the telephone rings you never know what you're going to get.

During my time as a vet a number of things have happened to me that I have never forgotten. In the pages of this book you will find weird and wonderful stories. Some are funny, some are heart-warming, some are painful; everything is true. The vast majority of them happened to me, though I have also included a few anecdotes that were told to me by colleagues. It is not a text book, so I have spared you a lot of the boring details, but I have, where possible, gone through patients' medical records for accuracy and interviewed some of the owners to fill in the gaps. I didn't have to dig for these stories, they're all seared into my memory and have been retold over many dinner tables. This book is a portrait of the first year of my life as an emergency vet.

Marc Abraham

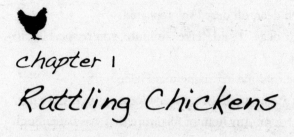

chapter 1
Rattling Chickens

Lack of sleep makes everything slow, it makes clocks and brains and bodies sluggish, and it makes it nigh on impossible to find anything good on television. In my years as an out-of-hours vet I found only one cure for sleepiness, the ringing telephone. Ours was one of those retro phones that looked like it was made of Bakelite. If we were going to be woken by a ringtone, we made sure it was a classy one.

'Good evening, surgery.'

I rolled the last 'r' in 'surgery' unintentionally. After weeks of business plans and paperwork, meetings with the practice's partners, and meetings about more meetings, Ruth, my nurse, and I had finally established the emergency vet service that Brighton had so desperately needed. We had been up and running for ten or so days and we were still feeling our way along.

'Oh dear,' said a husky woman's voice on the end of the line.

Of all the possible greetings, that isn't one you want to hear.

'Oh dear, oh dear,' she repeated.

'It's okay,' I said, 'take a minute, you're speaking to the vet.'

She told me her name was Helen.

As she went into what was wrong, my eyes did a tour of the room. Any item of furniture that was flat enough was topped with greetings cards. 'Good Luck on your new job', read one, sitting high on the filing cabinet. 'Don't muck it up', read its neighbour. Our futuristic new LCD television blared unfuturistic 80s music videos – The Police, Genesis, Paula Abdul. Over the hundreds of nights in front of us, the television would serve as a crude stressometer. When it was on, it meant that all was calm; when it was off, we were all systems go. I gestured to Ruth, who was standing by, to turn the volume down. The caller was noticeably agitated. She huffed and puffed into the phone as she spoke. Her words came out chopped up.

'I'm in ever such a flap,' she said, 'I don't know what's happened to chickens.'

I paused and took a breath.

'To who?'

'To chickens,' she said.

'Chickens?' I said, making triply sure I'd heard her right.

I waved at Ruth.

The television went off.

Over the next few minutes I asked Helen the best questions I could think of and listened in hard to her answers. I pressed the receiver into my ear to help suck some clarity out of what she was saying. I flapped at Ruth for a scrap of paper, and fished in my pockets for a ballpoint pen. I had a crib sheet on the desk with some instructions. Take their name. I jotted down *Helen*. Who's the patient? *Chickens*, question mark, exclamation mark. It all went down. The next prompt was to ask what the problem was. Everything to date had been reasonably routine, and in most cases you can triage easily over the phone. Not this one.

'He *what* when he walks? Rattles?'

I stared at the A4 print-out that was Blu-tacked to the wall – '*An emergency to you is an emergency to us.*' I suppose you could call it our ethos. It was also the first thing I'd ever laminated. There was a wrinkle right through the middle.

'Why don't you pop down,' I said, 'and we'll take a look.'

Ruth was an excellent nurse. When I interviewed her she had jet-black, punky hair down to her shoulders and an infectious optimism that Victor Meldrew would struggle to resist. When we first met she was wearing a Peruvian poncho, for her interview no less, and seemed unfazed by the panel of partners and a cynical head nurse. Fresh from six months back-packing in Latin America she had a tan like a wood-stained bodybuilder, and an air of unshakeable confidence. Her tan had faded in the three weeks since we hired her but her confidence remained. People have assumed that since Ruth and I get on so well there must be something between us. Well, there's not – we're just too different. And besides, Ruth is very happily ensconced in a quirky little flat with her boyfriend Rich.

'Who was that?' she asked, cradling a cup of ginseng tea in her hands.

My head was attending more immediate concerns. I peered over the rim of the mug. Half-drunk Nescafé. It looked like a muddy puddle.

'We urgently need a coffee machine,' I said.

I opened the fridge. Horror of horrors. How could we be out of milk already? I slammed the door shut. Then out of my mouth came three words that no self-respecting coffee-lover should ever have to put in sequence.

'Black Gold Blend?'

Ruth shook an Evian bottle of pale yellow liquid at me. She had a cute manner of talking. The end of every one of her sentences went up as if she was asking a question. It meant I nodded after everything she said, it was impossible not to.

'Beyoncé Diet,' she said, 'it's like a lemon cleanse?'

I nodded but I had no idea what she was talking about.

The back room of the surgery faced the car park. If you sat on the kitchen counter you looked out over the tarmac. Some nights we'd have back-to-back drop-ins and all the parking spaces would be full, on other nights we were like firemen between the sirens, wiling away the hours with crossword puzzles and MTV. There'd be nothing in the car park but a carrier bag rolling along in the wind. It was midnight. I stood at the window and watched for Helen through the slats of the blind. It was February and the rain had set in, and not a little drizzle either. It was the sort of weather you see in commercials for hug-in-a-mug soups and hot chocolates; theatrical flashes of lightning, rumbles of thunder and a downpour that stuck fringes onto foreheads. I swilled a mouthful of bitter instant coffee. I had nightmarish visions of Helen pulling up in a van or a lorry, stacked from the floor to the ceiling in hundreds of cages each occupied by a flapping bird. In my ten professional years so far I hadn't come across a single chicken, except, maybe between slices of bread. Then ten days into my own surgery and – BAM!

A pair of headlights bumped into the car park. The headlights didn't belong to a chicken lorry but to an old, blue Volvo. The front door swung open and into a puddle stepped a tatty pair of sports shoes. The woman who climbed out of the car had brown curly hair that was being drenched by the rain. She quickly hopped out of the puddle and in front of the headlights, turning her body into a silhouette. I opened the back door and called to her as the rain drummed on the flat roof.

'Do you want a hand bringing them in?' I shouted across the car park.

'Them?' she said.

There was a bark from the boot of her car.

'The birds?'

Helen fell quiet.

We swapped confused expressions for a moment.

'Birds?' she said.

She made her way towards me.

'Birds?' she said again, with an almost laugh, 'Do you mean Chickens?'

'Chickens' was a golden retriever.

Ruth led the way through the back door into the consulting room. In the professional surroundings of the surgery, I saw Helen's shoulders visibly relax. Ruth took her overcoat and hung it up on a hat-stand in the waiting room, then disappeared to put on the kettle. I passed Helen a paper towel to wipe the rain out of her eyes. Chickens, a beautiful ten-month-old golden retriever puppy, didn't look happy. He waddled into the room, and hunched by the table, bowing his head over his feathery chest, looking for all the world as if he was in prayer.

'He's been doing this since we came in from our walk,' said Helen, nervously scrunching the paper towel I gave her in her hand, 'and he comes down on his front legs like he's praying.'

She pressed her palms flat together as if uttering one of her own, then went back to scrunching the paper towel.

'Is he off his food?' I asked.

I looked up and saw Helen with her glasses off. Her wide eyes looked frazzled. She looked like a little girl sitting on the teacher's chair at school. Without her coat she looked small and pensive and she sat with her hands open in her lap, palms facing up to the ceiling. If I was to guess her occupation, I'd have gone for librarian. She nodded her head as she wiped her steamy spectacles with an ear of her polo shirt.

'He's been in his bed most of the day,' she said softly, 'I got him up, he did a couple of steps, then he does this...'

She leant forward and moved her hands by her throat to suggest he was retching.

'...but nothing comes out.'

Unproductive attempts to vomit, I noted to myself.

'Then I noticed when he started to walk that he made this rattling sound.'

She looked down at Chickens standing there.

'He's not doing it now. I'll tell you what it sounded like.'

She got a set of keys out of her bag and bashed them against the counter. The key fob was a plastic figurine of a cartoon character and the key ring was drilled through his feet. She silenced the jangling keys and rat-a-tat-tatted the plastic head against the countertop.

'No, that's not it.'

She furrowed her brow.

Helen reached for Chicken's collar and gave him a little tug. The retriever stumbled forwards.

'It's fine, Helen,' I said. 'Is he passing faeces?'

But she wouldn't let me finish. She walked him around the room. At first I heard nothing, but by the fifth or sixth step there was an audible sound. A faint clunk, clunk clunk, coming from his stomach.

'It's like salt pots bashing together,' she said.

I nodded as if I had some idea what that sounded like.

'Is he passing faeces?' I asked again.

'Is he?' she said. 'No, I don't think so.'

Chickens stopped and looked around, then stretched his neck and licked his sore stomach. Ruth gave Helen a mug of black tea and helped her to a seat while I put on my gloves and knelt down beside her dog.

'Will you hold his backside?' I said.

Helen put the mug down on the floor and stretched forwards.

I ran my fingers under his belly and felt about his abdomen. No sooner was I on my knees in order to examine him further, Chickens turned his head around and tried to grab the stem of my stethoscope, almost puncturing the thick rubber piping with his needle sharp teeth.

'Not for you,' I said, tucking it into my scrubs.

'He'll eat anything,' said Helen.

I got back to examining his abdomen. My fear was that this could be a gastric torsion, the 'golden emergency scenario', that would have been a real test after being open for just a few days. I threw a glance at Ruth; she looked worried. I ran my hand over his tender belly. At first everything felt fine, but then towards the back of his stomach, the part we call the caudal aspect, there was a bump, and then another, and one more. The stomach was protruding beyond the rear of the ribcage. Each lump was hard and spherical, each was a similar size, and when I pressed them, the patient whimpered. Helen was following everything I was doing, her eyes went wide like saucers. I put my stethoscope in my ears and pressed the chest piece onto his stomach. I find that a stethoscope can sometimes be more of a thinking device than anything else. It bought me some time to consider the options.

'It feels like there's something in his stomach,' I said.

'What?' she said. 'What is it? Is it bad? Is it awful? Tell me it's not bad.'

'I think he's eaten something he shouldn't. What I'll

do is perform an X-ray and then we'll be able to assess the situation.'

The X-ray took a while to perform. It was a conscious X-ray, which has the advantage of not having to use sedation, so it's usually both quicker and safer but with a lively puppy like Chickens it can be a fairly testing procedure as it relies on the patient lying still on the plate, not something that came easily to Chickens.

'He's a livewire, isn't he, Helen?' I said, as Ruth clipped the X-ray onto the light box.

Helen nodded. She was understandably tense.

I walked over to the light box and flicked the switch. The neon tube behind it flickered on. Foreign body ingestion can usually be easily confirmed with an X-ray depending on what the swallowed object actually is. Hard dense objects like bone or metal show up much better than softer objects like rubber or plastic. This one was very clear. Imagine shining a torch back at you through a big balloon, a balloon that contained a bunch of black grapes. There was a cluster of black circles, each one larger than a fifty pence piece. They were clustered at the base of the stomach.

'Oh no!' she said. 'Oh dear!'

'Helen, can I ask you a question?'

She nodded.

'Do you live near a golf course?'

*

Pre-med, propofol injectable anaesthetic, intravenous drip and in we go. We positioned Chickens on his back, fast asleep, with his legs tied down. It was straight through the mid-line to his stomach to perform a gastrostomy, literally a hole in his stomach to remove the offending items. Two and half hours on the operating table and 67 stitches. I thought he might have swallowed three or four of them but when we opened him up there were *nine* golf balls, turned brown by the acid in his stomach. It was unbelievable. Each golf ball was four centimetres in diameter and weighed close to two ounces. I had never seen anything remotely close to that size in a dog's stomach. With over a pound of them rattling around in his stomach it was no wonder Chickens was praying. I repaired the gastric wall with a couple of layers of inverting sutures, flushed the abdominal cavity with a few drip-bags worth of warm saline, and Chickens came round from his anaesthetic very smoothly. After a night in the hospital with Ruth and I desperately trying to stop him chewing his drip out of his leg using combinations of buster collars and more bandages, and then keeping down small portions of chicken and rice over the next 24 hours, he was collected by his whole family, and went home.

When I arrived at the surgery the following day there was a bunch of flowers waiting for me. The receptionist had cut their stems and left them standing in the kitchen sink. On the front, written in black fountain pen, was a little yellow card. 'Good luck with the new surgery.' I flipped it over. There wasn't a name, but there was something else written on the back – 'Don't count your Chickens before they've hatched.' I smiled to myself as I pinned the card to the corkboard in the common room. I had a feeling I'd see him again soon.

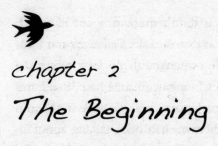

chapter 2
The Beginning

The day I resigned from my previous job is a day I shall never forget. I should be grateful that in my case, nerves manifest in punctuality rather than sweaty palms or worse, sweaty underarms. I arrived outside the surgery before it opened so I sauntered off to a newsagent's to buy a quarter of sherbet lemons.

I'd run that day through my head so many times I was in danger of being over-rehearsed. I had a fantasy of how it would play out. My eyes open at seven o' clock as the alarm clock slowly fades in. The curtains part to beautiful rays of sunlight, an aerial display team whizzes by, spelling out *Go Marc!* in a trail of coloured smoke. A bird flies through my window and lands on top of the radio. She pecks at the digital presets, and nudges the volume bar with her beak. Out of the speakers play the opening bars of 'What a Wonderful World', then Louis Armstrong's unmistakeable voice comes in. I arise from my bed refreshed and alert, ready to face the day with a smile on my face and a spring in my step.

Needless to say it didn't quite pan out like that. I didn't get so much as a wink of sleep all night and I was still tossing and turning when my alarm clock radio came to life with a blast of Chumbawumba. I had 33 minutes to get to work. It was January, and we were in the grip of winter. The weathermen had been talking about an icy blast that was blowing straight in from the Arctic, and everything had iced over, the roads, the cars and the pavements. I picked the thickest warmest jumper I could find in my chest of drawers. When I put it on it went up to my chin and stretched down to my knees, it resembled a hand-me-down from a professional wrestler. I have no idea where, when, or why I had bought it, but at least I was warm. I put on my winter gloves, laced up some pretty serious boots and set off on my mission to resign, looking like I was trekking to the North Pole.

Brighton is a large town with a two-legged population of about 150,000. At the time there were several veterinary practices but there was little provision for out-of-hours vets. I'd worked in clinics with them before, one in Cardiff and another a few miles down the road, and had seen first-hand how it could transform a business. Brighton was crying out for an emergency service that ran on nights and weekends, but however many times I tried, I could not convince my employers of the benefits of extending the surgery's remit. So I took the idea somewhere else. For four weeks I talked with another practice. The partners' names were George and Edward, though I had listed them as 'Brandy' and 'Stella' in my phone so as not to arouse suspicion should someone glance at my phone display. We held a series of secret meetings a few miles away in the wood and leather environment of the Sportsman's Bar at the Withdean Stadium. Judging by the other people in the room no one would have suspected we were having anything more than a friendly chat.

Not everyone, though, had a three-foot map. I arrived with one rolled-up under my arm, decorated with hundreds of stickers and different lengths of string. We unrolled it on a low bar table and I got to work explaining the plans. There were distances marked off in pencil, and numbers and figures dotted around on little white tabs: clusters of vets, numbers of nurses and case-load estimations. Over the weeks we worked through a careful business plan, a Word document that had started life as a few strokes on the back of a napkin, and shuttled back and forth between our computers. After three or four meetings we formally shook hands, and nine days later they'd re-jigged a few filing cabinets in their premises to make room for myself and a nurse.

It was the Monday team meeting and we'd reached that point in the agenda where the real discussions happen.

'Any other business?'

These words were normally my cue to come out of hibernation, but today I'd been paying careful attention and checking off the agenda points. We'd already reviewed the events of the past week, and discussed what was coming up in the next. The senior partner had read a note from someone who had asked to remain anonymous, 'Could we make sure we wash up our own mugs and not just leave them in the sink?' And then it was on to the AOBs. I suppose I could have taken the senior partner to one side, but I wanted all the partners to be there.

'I'm resigning,' I said, 'effective immediately.'

The three partners were sitting around in an arc like a council of wizards, arranged round me on comfy chairs with their knees up by their faces. 'You are?' said the senior partner with a note of surprise, his eyebrows curling upwards. I passed over my envelope, which was addressed to the three of them. The head nurse made a tiny cough, mumbled something under her breath, and scuttled out of the door. I looked from one partner to another, and found nothing but blank expressions on their faces.

'Any response?' I said.

On a human level, the partners and I came from different places. I was well travelled, impulsive and energetic; they were older than me, had never left Sussex, were happy with the status quo and disapproved of my

flip-flops. It was on my third week that I found an anonymous envelope sitting on top of my bag that contained a
photocopied page of my employment contract, the
section entitled *appropriate dress*. The words 'no pierc-
ings' had been highlighted. Perhaps life would have been
easier if I'd succumbed to a sports blazer and tie.

'Well,' I said, 'if that's all, can I just say thank you for
the, er, good times we've had.'

The council of wizards nodded. The senior partner
opened his mouth as if to say something, then stopped.
It was five weeks since I'd held showdown talks in the
very same room. Five weeks since I told them I wanted
to settle in Brighton but I wanted to be more than just
a long-term locum. Five weeks since one by one they
told me 'you're too immature', 'no one wants to work
with you', and 'you don't know the first thing about
business'.

I started to get up from my chair, then stalled.

'Oh, one more thing,' I said. 'From next week, I'm
starting an out-of-hours surgery up the road.'

The wizards fell out of their seats.

That night I telephoned my parents.

'Hi, Dad, I've got some news,' I said. 'Is Mum
around?'

Our family home is in Stanmore, north-west
London. My parents still live there. My dad, Tony, used

to work in advertising; amongst his achievements he was involved in the creation of Tony the Tiger, the chief spokesman for sugary cereals. My mum worked for the NHS, helping to repair the damage Dad caused.

'Jean,' Dad yelled with his mouth still next to the receiver. Not only did this nearly deafen me, but I'm sure every Jean in East Sussex stopped what they were doing and looked around. In the background my mother yelled back, 'I'll use the upstairs phone.' There were three in the house, all wired to different rooms. I had tried to introduce my parents to cordless phones but Mum kept taking the handsets to work. 'I've seen everyone else do it,' she said. I bit my tongue and got her a mobile for Christmas.

'Hello, love,' she said, joining in from the bedroom.

'He's got some news for us,' said Dad, in an ominous tone.

'Oh, you're not back with Steph, are you?' said Mum.

'Hang on,' I said. 'No I'm not.'

'It's not Kerry?' she said.

'No it's not, let me speak.'

'Let him speak,' said Dad.

'I was only asking,' said Mum.

I waited for the two of them to settle down. This bickering was part and parcel of domestic conference calls. Finally, there was a break in the conversation.

'I'm starting my own surgery,' I said.

There was a deafening silence. When they'd regained control of their tongues, they both talked at the same time so it just came out as a jumbled 'What did you say?'

I took a breath.

'I've left,' I said. 'I'm starting a new out-of-hours surgery up the road with another practice. It's all agreed with the partners.'

'Are you joking?' said Mum.

'Is this a wind-up?' asked Dad. 'How many places have you worked at now? Five?'

'I thought you'd be thrilled,' I said.

'What's happened this time?'

A ball of tumbleweed rolled past, made up of every parent–child disagreement we'd ever had. I felt my shoulders sink into my body. It was as if I was ten years old all over again. What followed was a spirited five-minute defence of my decision from me, then a twenty-minute argument, which concluded in a very detailed character assassination from my father charting the eight years from university to now. Mum bowed out after ten minutes telling me that whatever I choose to do she'd support me, and then she calmly put down the phone.

Dad continued his rant. 'Well, here's something you need to think about – it's called settling down, Marc.'

'Thank you, Dad,' I said, 'I'm sure I will.'

We parted on those words. I rocked back in my chair. *It could have been worse*, I thought to myself, *I could have had Dad down as a reference.*

chapter 3
Teething Problems

The new practice was a breath of fresh air. There was still a faint whiff of conservatism but it was countered by an energy and a desire to do right by the animal and its owner. Ruth and I agreed it would be a good idea to arrive early for our first day. Neither of us had seen the space that they'd cleared for us and we didn't even know how the switchboard worked. I'd arranged with George, the senior partner, that we should have a proper induction; it was somehow pared back to a two-hour chat prior to our first shift.

I met Ruth in a greasy café across the street and quickly discovered that we had different methods of psyching ourselves up for the big day. I had made a careful and considered playlist for my iPod. The selection criteria was simple: 1) the energy levels should be high, 2) the embarrassment factor, if overheard on the bus, should be low and 3) it should be easy to sing to. By these principles 'Eye of the Tiger' was in and 'My Heart Will Go On' was most definitely out. Ruth's preparations were a little more New Age. When I turned the corner, head nodding to 'Ghetto Superstar' she was quietly meditating by an outside table over a eucalyptus tea. I quickly whipped out my earphones.

'Do they serve that here?' I said, wrinkling my nose. I looked from her thick woolly jumper to the Day-Glo starbursts plastering the window that yelled 'Kidney and chips' and 'Cappuccinos'. Ruth reached into her pockets and withdrew a polythene bag full of leaves and a few sachets of honey.

'I made my own,' she said, and pulled out a chair for me.

It had been one of those bright, clear winter days, but now as the clock ticked on to four, shadows lengthened and I was glad of my woollen hat that covered my shaven head. With our table overlooking the surgery, and clutching our hot drinks to keep our hands warm, we watched clients troop in and out. A lady came out with a cat carrier, a girl with a miniature Yorkshire terrier poking its head out of her handbag, a young boy struggling with a noisy cardboard box. It was just like every other surgery in every other town, there was nothing remotely remarkable about it. Aside from one thing: every evening, as soon as the clocked ticked past six, I was in charge.

'We should probably head over,' said Ruth.

She slurped the final mouthfuls of her strong-smelling tea.

*

Strange as it may seem, I had only been inside the surgery once before. It was a plain brick building with automatic doors and a fish tank in the waiting room; that was as much as I could remember. We weren't expecting balloons and 'WELCOME, MARC AND RUTH!' banners, but I think we both thought there'd be some sort of a reception when we walked up to the front desk. Nobody so much as looked up.

'Is it Gloria?' I asked the bouffant hair behind reception.

'Depends who's asking,' said its owner, her head very much in her work, filing something away in a folder.

'It's Marc,' I said, 'and Ruth.' I paused. 'We're due to meet George?'

Gloria froze. Her head came up and she looked us up and down as if inspecting prospective suitors for her daughter. Suddenly everything changed.

'Gloria,' she said, over the top of her reading glasses, and she held out her hand.

We made our introductions. Neither of us realised this at the time, but the sight of her face in the mornings would be like a glimpse of an approaching passenger ship to a desert island castaway. Gloria was a relief in every possible sense. We'd take the practice off her hands at six every night and hand it back to her at eight the next morning. Working weekends meant six o'clock Friday to eight o'clock Monday with no break in between. So on a Monday morning at eight o'clock, there was no word in the English language more welcome than *Gloria*. She was small and round and happy, and almost a stereotype of what it is to be Welsh. To be born Welsh, she would say, quoting Wilfred Wilson, was to be born privileged, not with a silver spoon in your mouth but with music in your blood and poetry in your soul.

Gloria led us through to the back room, where George and Edward were waiting.

'Marc! Ruth!' George cried, leaping to his feet, 'Welcome, welcome, welcome.'

George was the senior partner and had a habit of repeating words for effect. He was a warm man with a penchant for trying to spot the next generation of classic cars, which gave him an extraordinary collection of questionable relics and the odd Jaguar XJS. He and Edward were chalk and cheese. Edward, his partner, was quite possibly the most serious man I've met. He owned three calculators but not a single mobile phone.

Edward hung back by his chair while George came forward to hug us.

'How are you both? So good to see you, Ruth.'

George's eyes were smiling. We had an instant connection. You couldn't leave his company without feeling optimistic and energetic. And he couldn't remember the first thing about the 60s, which proved he was really there. By contrast, Edward was the leftovers of the

Victorian era jumbled into a middle-aged man, a fantastic bubble-and-squeak of waistcoats and formal manners. He was tall, intelligent and stiff. He wore a watch and starched his collars. I shook him formally by the hand.

'Well,' said George, 'let's give you the grand tour.'

We went on a ten-minute wander through a series of interconnected rooms. George insisted on leading the way like a hyperactive tour guide. No object escaped a remark.

'The kettle,' he said with a flourish, 'I imagine that will see some action.'

He looked at us expectantly; we gave him a small smile.

The tour party moved on to a door marked 'Necessarium' which housed a toilet and a basin.

'And now, the room we saved till last,' said George. He locked eyes with the pair of us. 'Your new home.'

As he uttered those words he flung open the door and semi-bowed. When he straightened up he made a sweep of his hand and showed off the room like a magician's assistant. Edward appeared behind him, looking characteristically dour. The space they had made available was for our own exclusive use. It was a room about three by three metres that had had many past lives, most recently a storage room, as the dusty pink carpet, a bright pink trim around the edge where archiving boxes had once sat, testified. There were no windows; the only light came from a pair of fluorescent tubes. The partners had moved in one desk, one swivel chair, one very low easy chair, and a military green filing cabinet. There was a wall chart calendar tacked to the wall. And that was it. Not exactly cosy, but it was fine for our needs.

'Thank you, guys,' I said, setting down my rucksack.

Four pairs of eyes peeled around the room looking for something that ought be said, or that needed to be done. There was a feeling in the air. The same feeling I got the day my parents dropped me off at Edinburgh University, unpacked my boxes from the car and set them down in my new room, before driving straight back to London.

Edward broke the silence.

'Well, I suppose we should leave you both to settle in. If you need anything, just ask,' he said, mechanically.

The partners smiled and shuffled out, pulling the door to behind them. Ruth and I swapped glances, then our eyes drifted over to the clock.

The out-of-hours surgery had been marketed throughout the practice with yellow flyers on the front desk and orange A4 print-outs on the pillars. The plan was to eventually serve all the practices in a 25-mile radius, dispensing advice, diagnosing pet problems and conducting emergency surgery if needed, but to start with we worked with a handful of local surgeries. I unzipped my bag and took out a couple of cards. One had a champagne cork blasting into the air with the word *Congratulations* written in its bubbly trail. Inside was my dad's unmistakable handwriting, 'Good luck, son, you're gonna be great,' and 'Don't say I didn't warn you,' which I'm sure he meant as a joke. Gloria popped her head round the door. We were both looking up at the wall.

'Oh, I should point out that the clock's a little slow,' she said, 'I think it loses about a minute a day. I don't know why we don't get it fixed but there you go.' She shook her head, then carried on, 'There's a stool in the kitchen if you need to reach the shelves. And a carrot cake in the fridge. Help yourself. And if you need me, I'm afraid I shan't be much help tonight.' She winked and pursed her lips together. 'I plan on getting sloshed,' she said.

And then she was gone, her shoes clopping down the corridor.

The clock on the wall was a plate with pictures of cats painted around the rim. There was a different breed occupying the position that a number would normally be. The second hand worked its way round to the top. We traced its last steps from a lilac British shorthair, 56, 57, 58, 59, to a Siamese. I raised my eyebrows. Ruth managed a heart-felt *hurray*. It was like New Year's Eve all over again. There was no singing or fireworks, but like

New Year's it was a teeny bit of an anticlimax. Nothing had changed and nothing was different. There weren't owners hammering at the doors. The phone switchboard didn't start flashing red. The phone didn't ring.

I rocked back in the swivel chair. 'And they're off,' I said, in a sports commentator voice. Ruth forced a smile. She was sitting on the easy chair. It was so laid back she was practically on the floor. It was as if we were two strangers on the most awkward date.

'Here's to us,' I said, raising an empty desk-tidy.

Ruth laughed, and raised an imaginary glass to me.

My eyes skirted around the room to find something else to comment on, but returned without finding anything funny. A minute hadn't even gone past. *So this is it, is it?* I thought to myself. Nervous energy coursed through my body and emerged in a bout of fidgets. My hands found the lever that operated the height of my seat. I plunged down towards the floor, snorted like a schoolboy, and pumped myself back up again. Within thirty seconds my fingers were off. I drummed my fingers on the desktop, then found a lump of chewing gum, stuck to the underside of the table, hard like plastic. I stared at the phone for two minutes straight, as if willing it into life. We'd barely been open five minutes and I was already wishing I'd brought my crossword book.

Ruth scrunched up her nose. 'How long d'you think before it rings?' she said.

I shrugged.

'But if it doesn't,' I said, 'we could take turns to call in and pretend.'

What's that noise? I woke up with a start, my bleary eyes peered around the room. I was slumped over the desk in a swivel chair, no idea what the time was. And then it went again. I stared at the grey plastic thing in front of me.

'Ruth!' I shouted. 'It's ringing!'

There was a squeal of delight from the kitchen, followed by the sound of Ruth's hurried steps down the corridor. *Take a breath, Marc. Keep calm*, I told myself and placed my hand on the receiver.

'Good evening,' I said, 'surgery.'

Ruth huddled round, wide-eyed with expectation.

Then a beery voice said, 'What's on specials?'

'Excuse me?' I said.

'We want one chicken korma, a balti, two pilau, two peshwari naans, and an aloo gobi.'

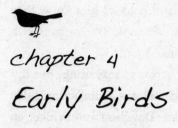

chapter 4
Early Birds

Our first proper patient arrived at a quarter past three.

'He's here!' Ruth yelled down the hall. 'I'll put the kettle on.'

To say it came as a relief would be an understatement. It had been nine hours since we had opened, and all we had to show for ourselves were five empty coffee mugs, a packet of Wotsits and Duran Duran Night on MTV. We'd talked until our mouths ached. We'd covered off our top ten music videos, the first singles we'd bought at Woolworths, we'd swapped embarrassing first-day-of-school anecdotes and tried to figure out if we had been in Bangkok at the same time. In nine hours the telephone had only rung three times, and two of those were for Indian takeaways. So whether this patient could have waited until the morning was neither here nor there, we weren't about to turn them away.

As soon as I saw the clients arrive I opened the door to the car park and began to walk out towards them, determined to show our first patients a warm reception. Anxious to convey the magnitude of their visit, I gripped the owner firmly by the hand, and let him know they were our first.

'We're night-shift virgins,' I said.

It may not have come across as reassuring, but this owner didn't seem to mind. Bill was a Hell's Angel. He had pulled up on a Harley Davidson motorbike, an immaculately polished silver and blue tourer. He took off his open-faced helmet and shook out his long silver hair as if we were shooting a shampoo commercial. On the back of his leather jacket was the famous winged skull logo and the slogan: HELLS ANGELS FOREVER. Bill had an unlikely passenger. On the back of the bike, at the end of the leather seat, secured with two yellow bungee cords, was a birdcage cloaked in a thick blanket.

'What's his name?' I said, lifting the cloth for a peek.

Bill looked me straight in the eye.

'Pretty Boy,' he said, without a trace of irony.

I nodded and swallowed a smile. Best to keep the 'pets look like their owners' joke to myself.

Pretty Boy was a beautiful green and yellow budgerigar and, just like a Norwich City football fan, he didn't have much to sing about. His head was tucked under his wing and his feathers fluffed out. Although budgerigars are usually healthy, robust creatures, they are susceptible to several minor ailments and few of a somewhat more serious nature. The floor of his cage was caked in diarrhoea.

These can be the tell-tale signs of enteritia, a condition caused by a run-down liver. Ruth greeted Bill with a steaming mug of tea and the four of us headed off down the corridor to the consulting room.

There were two consulting rooms in the surgery. They were roughly the size of a medium-sized bedroom in a terraced house. We went into Consulting Room 2. There were posters on the walls – 'PARASITE PROTECTION MADE EASY', a laminated diagram of a rabbit's digestive tract and another of feline dentition. There were weighing scales, a fridge, and a photo board with snaps of patients sent in by their owners.

I took my place behind the table and put on a pair of gloves. The strip-light flickered above me. An alien arriving from outer space would no doubt comment that everything in the room was green, from our clothes, to the walls, to the rope ties that held the curtains apart. Everywhere you went you met the same light green tone. Call me a geek, but I've researched its place in the medical world. Though the colour has long been associated with the feeling of calm, it wasn't always. It was first chosen by a psychiatrist in Philadelphia called Thomas Kirkbride, an architect of mental institutions in the nineteenth century. He introduced the colour on a rational whim because it signified growth, renewal and health. Playing devil's advocate green is also, I might add, the colour of money, jealousy and mushy peas. I've come to conclude that the psychology of colour isn't an exact science, but I digress.

Any vet will tell you that budgies are notoriously hard to hold, examine and medicate. They can become stressed very easily and it's not uncommon for them to suffer a fatal cardiac arrest when held by their vet or even their owner. So Ruth set about making the room as stress-free as possible. It was second nature to her. Without saying a word she dimmed the lights to a lower level, shut the door and made sure all the escape routes were closed. I was wearing rubber gloves to as to reduce the chances of cross infection. We were set. With a flip of a catch, I opened the cage, and took the bird in my fingers. Bill craned in to look. The budgie didn't object; enteritia usually makes a bird tame. Contrary to popular mythology – see 'bird-brained' in the dictionary – budgerigars are an intelligent species. So perhaps Pretty Boy knew where he was, and sensed that the fingers that were smoothing his feathers and untucking his head meant him no harm.

'Do you feed him anything other than seeds?'

Bill shook his head. 'Not really.'

Pretty Boy's fluffed-up appearance suggested that he'd been ill for over 24 hours. Luckily he was still drinking so his prognosis wasn't as guarded as other poorly budgies I'd examined before. I moved a cotton bud in front of him, which never usually fails to bring on a biting frenzy, but Pretty Boy didn't flicker. It was clear that he was deteriorating fast, and needed sorting out immediately. Ignoring a disease like enteritia can frequently be fatal.

'You don't feed him anything sugary or starchy? A lot of owners give them crisps,' I said, 'you know, as a treat every now and then.'

A little colour swept into Bill's face. He glanced at the floor.

'For other owners it's biscuits. Break the corner off a bourbon, poke it through the bars.'

Bill swung his motorcycle boot over the tiles, as if trying to shoe an invisible cat. Then he slowly lifted his face up.

'I, er, do give him the odd bite of cake,' he admitted, 'now and then.'

'Now and then?'

I had visions of the macho biker in a chintzy floral front room, pouring a cup of Darjeeling from a tea set complete with a cosy, and delicately cutting a budgie-sized pyramid of Battenberg with a cake fork.

'Well, perhaps more than I should.'

And there was the answer.

The cause of enteritia is an internal one, commonly by simply not feeding your budgie correctly with the right food like normal seed, but instead letting them eat 'junk food' titbits e.g. cake, potato and other such foods that are particularly sugary and starchy. This in turn causes the liver to be overtaxed, run down and results in awful diarrhoea.

It is difficult to find a good bird vet. The focus in vet schools has always primarily been on cats and dogs and large animal medicine. Unfortunately you hear stories of veterinarians 'winging it'. The majority of cases I see are routine and common conditions, but I will always call an avian specialist if something comes up that stumps me.

Ruth and I waved goodbye to Bill and Pretty Boy from the back step. Enteritia is simple enough to treat. I told Bill to cover three sides of the cage and sit him by the fire, letting him rest. And with a little bismuth carbonate sprinkled over his seed, he'd be chirping away in no time. Bill secured the birdcage back in place with the bungee cords, and with a low growl and a roar the happy couple in leather jacket and blanket disappeared off into the night.

Quarter to four. Four hours to go. We walked back through the labyrinth of interconnected rooms, the X-ray room, the operating theatre, the prep room, the in-patients' kennels. I suddenly became very conscious that the energy and banter that had characterised the first half of the night had slipped out of the back door when we let Bill and the budgie out. As we traipsed back to our office, the collective voices of all the doubters whispered in my head. My old nurse in my left ear, 'you'll never deal with the nights', the old partners in my right, 'too immature, too lazy, knows nothing about business'. And as I sat down by my desk and felt my head grow tired, I heard one all-too-familiar voice in the distance, 'You're not back with Steph, are you?' said my mother.

Gloria knew how to use her voice. She could make it as soft and as comforting as the shipping forecast on a sleepless night or as loud as a colliery band. This morning she chose the trumpet.

'Wakey, wakey, rise and shine,' her brassy, raspy tones travelled the short distance between her mouth and my sleeping ear. My body jerked violently awake. The small smiling face of Gloria was inches away from mine.

'Big night?' she said with a giggle.

I yawned and stretched out like a cat, and gave a grunty sigh.

'Was it busy?'

I lifted my head off the desk.

'We should get you a blanket,' she teased.

Gloria gave me the slightest pat on the shoulder then pottered off to the kitchen warbling away like her surname was Estefan. I knew she went to the kitchen because I heard the cabinet doors shut in-between snatches of 'I wanna dance with somebody'.

'You're hiding your hangover well,' I said, having followed her down the corridor.

'What d'you say?' she asked.

I walked to the counter and leant on it, watching Gloria as she started the washing up.

'You hide your hangover well,' I said.

'Well, I've had one or two years of practice,' she replied.

She popped in the plug and filled the sink.

'I'd better go wake up Ruth,' I said, wiping a fleck of dribble off my scrubs. I turned around to leave but when I got to the doorway I stopped.

'There is one thing,' I said. 'Do you get many phone-calls for Indian takeaways?'

Gloria looked at me curiously.

'Do *I* get people calling *me* for Indian takeaways?'

I nodded.

'No, just people wanting pizzas. I do a very good Hawaiian,' she said.

'Really?'

'No, of course not,' she replied, 'what are you talking about? Are you losing it, Marc?'

I didn't know how to answer that.

'Maybe,' I said, 'maybe.'

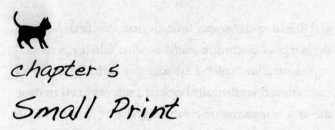

chapter 5
Small Print

Something strange happens when you drive into the
countryside. When you leave the smog of life behind and
disappear into hedgerows and green grassy fields that
spread for miles. When seagulls give way to pheasants
and bands of marauding students are swapped for flocks
of sheep. The South Downs is the most bewitching
stretch, a swathe of chalky land from Meon to Beachy
Head, with cliffs and hills, gorse and sapphire sea.

The taxi driver turned his head. 'Even on the dullest
days you never get tired of it,' he observed. I nodded,
yawning in the back.

As we wound our way towards Newhaven, the words
of William Henry Hudson seemed to whistle through
the gap in the driver's window, 'the ground never rises
above eight hundred and fifty feet, but we feel on top of
the world.' I'm sorry, Mr Hudson, but on four hours'
sleep and two Marmite crumpets, I'd have to disagree.

This journey was business not pleasure. We were
on our way to Seaford. No late-night pet surgery can
operate without wheels for the odd house visit, so Ruth

and I had spent some time during our first night in the surgery circling classifieds with felt-tip pens and copies of *Autotrader*. Fast forward eight hours and I had rather optimistically booked a one-way taxi to drop me at a bungalow on Seaford seafront, where a man called Alan had a Fiat Cinquecento that he'd listed in the Bargains section.

FIAT CINQUECENTO. RED 3-DOOR HATCH. ALTHOUGH
160,000 MILES, ENGINE SWEET. BODYWORK NOT
PERFECT BUT DOES HAVE YEAR'S MOT. RADIO.
REAR WASH/WIPE. HATED REAR WINDSCREEN.
£395 ONO. CALL ALAN

When I called Alan I forgot to ask if 'hated rear windscreen' was a typo, or whether he had something against them.

Alan was a little round man. Retired. Ex-postmaster. Bodywork not perfect, he walked with a cane. The wind was blowing strong and as he stepped out of the door, his thin white hair blew up like sea grass in the dunes.

'It's my wife's car,' he said, gesturing to a shadowy figure watching from behind the net curtains. 'Or it was,' he revealed. 'We let the grandkids use it. That was a mistake.'

We took two full laps of the car. The 'hated rear windscreen' seemed to be a typo, rather than how Alan felt about the car's back window. He crouched to show me some rust around the wheel arches.

'As I said, we've not had any problems, but the sea air isn't great, what with all the salt in it.'

You can never be sure what multitude of sins are pardoned by expressions like 'bodywork not perfect' but when I lifted the boot I could see straight through to the drive.

'Ooh,' I said, tracing my finger around the rim of a hole.

We walked around to the driver's door. The envelope containing eight fifty-pound notes was burning a hole in my pocket. I sunk my hand in and held it; the feel of a wad of real money helps to focus the mind. Every car I've ever owned has been cursed. It's not that I'm technically inept, nor that I have an allergy to grease. I'm unlucky. My first car gave up the ghost on the way to a surfing weekend in Wales. Needless to say, marooned on the hard shoulder of the M4 our surfboards never saw the sea. The second car, an ancient Rover, joined the great scrapheap in the sky in slippery conditions in Bracknell. It took the local fire brigade to remove it from the wall of the leisure centre car park. So as I sank into the rather spongy front seat of Alan's car, I checked the rear-view mirror for black cats.

'It has had some knocks,' said Alan, 'but it goes like a dream.'

'What sort of dream?' I asked.

He laughed with me and not in a reassuring way.

*

My mother is a helpaholic, that is, she is one of those people who 'just wants to help' even when uninvited, no, especially when uninvited. She's been this way for as long as I can remember, but her disorder spiralled out of control when Dad introduced her to something called Google. Nowadays you must be very careful what you say. Should a careless word escape from your lips, you'll hear her fingers tapping. 'Brazil-tropical-diseases' then hit return; 'Safety-motorbikes' return; 'jet-ski accidents' return. I'd always considered myself a night-owl, so I wasn't daunted by the prospect of working through the night, but my boasting to Mum on the way back from Seaford that, like Margaret Thatcher, my body worked fine on three hours' sleep, was bravado mixed with idiocy. In my defence, I was tired. I arrived home to seven emails. Aside from the one offering cheap Viagra, they were all from my mother. I opened the first.

From: Mum
Date: Tuesday, 5 February, 1:23 pm
To: Marc
Subject: CONCERNING

Marc,

After our chat about the job, I've done a little research. Speaking to Dad as well we are both

worried. I found this article you should read –
'Doctor falls asleep in surgery'. It was posted on
April 16th by Medical Negligence. Quite sobering.
Maybe you and your nurse should think about
sleeping in shifts like they do in the Navy?

Love Mum.

I clicked on the next one.

From: Mum
Date: Tuesday, 5 February, 1:29 pm
To: Marc
Subject: Re: CONCERNING

Marc,

Just found this:
Shift work sleep disorder from Wikipedia, the free
encyclopedia.
Shift work sleep disorder (SWSD) is a circadian
rhythm sleep disorder which affects people who
change their work or sleep schedules frequently.

Such recurrent interruption of sleep patterns may
result in insomnia and/or excessive sleepiness. A
2007 study led by the IARC (International Agency for

Research on Cancer) showed that shift work can
induce cancer.

Ignore my bit in the previous email about the Navy.
Your auntie reminded me of something your
granddad used to say. 'You cannot skip sleep, you
can only borrow against it.'

Mum.

I rolled my eyes at a third, sent ten minutes later, entitled 'Tips on how to stay awake'. It appeared to be the
contents of a webpage that she had copied-and-pasted
without reading all the way down. The advice was
given by an American man who claimed to have kept
himself awake for seven days straight. Was this proof of
the efficacy of his tips or evidence of lunacy? Suggestions included water, bright lights, and fresh air, all
common sense, then tip number seven: listen to a
Christian rock station. Tip eight was Ben and Jerry's
Chunky Monkey. I returned to my inbox, highlighted
the block of messages from my mother and sent them
to the trash, with a mumbled apology. Just as I was
about to turn it off a new message pinged in. This time
from Dad.

From: Dad
Date: Tuesday, 5 February, 4:17 pm
To: Marc
Subject: Mrs T

Marc,

Not sure Margaret Thatcher was the best example
of someone who looks good on little sleep. Are you?

Dad

chapter 6
The Cat Who Laid an Egg

We'd barely hung up our coats when the practice phone rang. Day two. It was chucking it down outside again and the thick donkey jacket I'd been wearing didn't offer much in the way of protection. I don't know whether my mother's nerves had got to me, but I arrived much more prepared today. Like an eager boy scout I emptied the contents of my rucksack onto the shelf in the changing room – a couple of cans of Red Bull next to Ruth's packet of herbal marshmallow cigarettes, front-line ammunition in the battle to stay on top. Both cans were for me, one for mid-way through the evening, the other only if I hit 'the wall'. Ruth wasn't going to be joining me. When I showed up in the red Fiat Cinquecento, she was already in the kitchen whisking up her own natural energy booster, two tablespoons of ground thyme steeped in hot water. I had taken off my trainers and was putting on my rubber clogs when she knocked on the door and entered without waiting for an answer.

'Marc, will you speak to this lady?'

Ruth's expression screamed 'urgent', so I fastened up my scrubs as we tripped down the corridor. Ruth leant against the doorframe as I took a seat in the office. The phone receiver was lying on the desk. I took a little breath and turned in my chair so that I could read Ruth's face and so she could see mine. The caller was Portuguese. Not only did she have a thick Latin accent but also a limited English vocabulary. She ended each sentence with my name – 'Mr Abraham' – and her intonation rose as if she was pleading with me.

'She's howling?' I said.

'Can you hear it, Mr Abraham?'

The lady held the phone up so I heard nothing for a while, then came a low, whiney yowl.

'Did you hear it, Mr Abraham?' she said again, 'She pacing, pacing, pacing. Up and down. Up and down.'

'Is she pregnant?' I asked.

There was a pause on the end of the line.

'She is tortoise.'

'Tortoise?' I asked.

'Tortoise cat,' she said.

'No, I meant, is she pregnant, er, is she going to have kitten babies?' I asked.

'Maybe,' she said. 'How can they tell, Mr Abraham?'

It's not uncommon for owners not to notice that their pet is pregnant until very late on.

'She is fat,' she said, 'she is very fat. I kneel down, Mr Abraham.'

I listened as the owner knelt on the floor beside her cat. There was clunk as the receiver knocked against the floor. She held the phone close to the cat so I could hear a rhythmical purring.

'That's good,' I said.

'Oooh,' said the lady, 'she's making milk.'

There are many signs that a cat is about to give birth. Typical signs can include anxious restless behaviour as she searches for a place to kitten. Vigilant owners will monitor the cat's temperature too, as approaching birth it will usually drop by a degree or so from normal. I think the penny must have dropped because I heard her squeal.

'Oh my *God*! Mr Abraham,' she said. 'Oh my GOD!' The kitten bombshell had just exploded across the phone-lines.

'It's fine,' I said. 'Why don't you sit down?'

I coached her over to her kitchen chair.

'Are you okay?' I asked.

She was jittering with a cocktail of emotions, two parts fear to one part excitement. She had been difficult to understand at the beginning of the conversation but now I was having trouble letting her know what she should do. I spoke very slowly.

'Have you had cats before?' I asked.

'No, Mr Abraham, is neighbour's,' she said.

'Is your neighbour there?' I asked.

Ruth's eyes went wide as she tried to make sense of things from only hearing one side of the conversation. She played with her hair, twirling it around a finger.

'No, Mr Abraham, is away,' said the lady.

'He's away?' I said. 'For how long?'

I think I expected her to tell me they'd popped out for a pint of milk or were away for a day or two.

'For six months,' came her reply. 'How do I make babies come?'

I could understand her panic. This was not her area of expertise. I learned later that the lady's neighbour was a marketing consultant and had been sent by his company to work in their big office in Philadelphia. He was understandably wary about taking his cat to a foreign country, especially when he had to be working so much and travelling round the East Coast so he had asked her if she would mind cat-sitting. It turned out that she had only been doing this for a month, and never having looked after a cat before was coming across a whole new set of experiences. I tried to reassure her that problems during pregnancy and birth in cats are pretty rare in all breeds apart from Persians perhaps, and usually most moggies deliver their kittens without assistance or complications.

'Best thing is not to disturb her,' I said, 'give her some space. But maybe leave the door open so you can monitor things.'

The cat was undoubtedly fine; it was the poor cat-sitter I was worried about.

'How long should I wait?' she asked.

Ruth went outside to greet a dog owner that had arrived in the car park while I explained the full ins and outs of the birthing process to the Portuguese cat-sitter, letting her know what to expect so there weren't any further surprises. I talked her through everything, how the first kitten should arrive within an hour after the onset of labour, and how sometimes labour lasts only a few minutes before the kitten arrives.

'Other kittens should arrive with an interval of ten minutes to an hour between them,' I said. 'Everything should be fine, but call me if you have any trouble.'

Our second night could not have been more different to the first. Patients were in and out of the surgery as if a neon sign had been planted in the car park. Either Gloria had been doing a hard sell or word was quickly spreading, in any case our phone did not stop from 6 pm till midnight.

We saw another budgie, this time with a feather cyst.

We saw a beautiful black Labrador called Sparky who, catching a whiff of a rabbit, had dived under a Land Rover and opened a three-inch wound along his back. I shaved a five-by-two inch rectangle of fur from around the wound, much to the proud owner's chagrin, and tidied up fresh edges to make a clean stitch. The owner in Barbour jacket and wellington boots complimented my 'nice piece of embroidery' and suggested that next time I should shave something cool into his fur, like 'Paws Rock!'

We had a dog called Odie, who'd been rubbing his bottom along the carpet. He had an anal gland that desperately needed emptying.

We had a cat that had eaten his sister's biscuits and suffered an allergic reaction. Harry was one of those cats that ate anything he could find, and it was a full-time job for his owners to make sure that he only ate the food that was for him. He had skin lesions right the way down his back that he scratched with his hind paws until they were red raw. I clipped and cleaned the area and applied an ointment before wrapping his back feet in bandages to stop it getting any worse. It came as a shock for Harry, who slipped around the treatment table like a foal on an ice rink.

All evening Ruth and I worked flat out, there had been no time for a Red Bull or a herb-and-hot-water break.

'She's on the phone again,' said Ruth.

'Who?' I said.

'The Portuguese woman,' she said.

Ruth passed me the phone. I hadn't even got it up to my ear before she asked, 'Mr Abraham. Can I poke finger in her?'

I was taken aback.

'*No*,' I said, 'absolutely not. Leave her where she is. Are there any kittens yet?'

'No,' said the lady. 'She move to the bedroom, Mr Abraham. I follow her from a distance and spy on her.'

'Where are you now?' I asked.

'Outside the bedroom, you tell me not to disturb so I close the door, shall I open?' she said.

'I imagine she was just looking for a nice warm place to have them,' I said. 'Don't take it personally but she'd probably rather you weren't around. But it's okay to have a peek and check on things.'

'Can I now?' she asked.

'Go on,' I said, 'I'll stay on the line.'

I heard the door creak open, and then it went quiet for a minute. Then there was a gasp, the sound of the phone dropping to the carpet and an ear-piercing screech. It was a long-held note that lasted for a few seconds. She was no longer holding the phone but I could still hear her.

'There's an egg, Mr Abraham, I see an EGG!' she said.

When she picked up the receiver again I tried to calm her down.

'Sssshh,' I said, 'you'll frighten her.'

'It's an *egg*,' she said hysterically, 'an egg. Oh. MY. GOD. There isn't a baby inside.'

'It's a placenta,' I said firmly.

'No,' she said, 'an egg.'

I was wondering whether I'd have to explain to her that cats do not lay eggs, as far as I know there are only three mammals that do – the platypus, the short-beaked echidna and the long-beaked echidna (also known as spiny anteaters). But she didn't want a biology lesson.

'Oh. MY. *GOD*,' she said.

'It's a placenta.'

'An *egg*,' she said. 'There isn't a baby inside.'

We toed and froed for a couple of minutes, but she simply wouldn't have it.

'An *EGG*, Mr Abraham!' she insisted.

'Don't panic,' I said finally, 'have you got a car?'

Ruth and I couldn't leave the surgery in busy periods and struggling to know what else to say I invited her in to see me with both the mother and her 'egg'.

We stood in the car park like a pair of naughty teenagers. Ruth was half-in, half-out the back door so she could have one of her marshmallow cigarettes and listen for the phone. I sat on the step. She'd offered me one, but I'm more the fresh-air type.

'I can't believe you bought that heap of crap,' she said, signalling the red Cinquecento.

'I can't believe you're smoking a marshmallow,' I said.

'It's marshmallow herb, rose petal and clover. Totally non-addictive. No nicotine, no tobacco. Smooth and satisfying,' she said. 'So there.'

'I just don't get you sometimes, Ruth,' I said. 'It's a mystery we get along as well as we do. And next time you laugh at my car, just remember that you were the one who spotted it.'

'As a joke,' she said, taking another deep drag of her herbal cigarette and blowing a stream of sugary-smelling smoke into the night air. 'Well, I'm not going on a visit in that! We'd *never* make it back.'

'She's a fine little car,' I said loyally.

'She's a load of junk.'

I pulled a disappointed face. 'Ruth, how could you? Cars have feelings too. If you can't say it to her face…'

Before I could finish the sentence, Ruth left her sentry post and walked up to the bonnet. She crouched down by the front grille, and stroked the Fiat badge.

'You're a no-good piece of crap,' she whispered, 'but I love you.'

We laughed so hard we went red in the face.

'What a mad old night!' I said.

'And it's only day two,' she said.

Ruth scrunched her cigarette out under her trainers. She looked at me with one of those looks women sometimes make, where they screw up their eyes a bit and their brow becomes furrowed, and they just look at you and wait for you to ask.

'What?' I said.

'Why don't you have a girlfriend?' she said.

'A girlfriend? I'm too much for one girl to handle. I need a whole staff to tend my needs...'

'I'm being serious,' said Ruth.

'So am I,' I said, 'sort of. I dunno, why do *you* think?'

'You really want to know what I think?' she said.

'Yes,' I replied.

'Sure?'

I nodded.

'All right then, Marc,' she said, 'here's what I think. I think you've got a short attention span. I think you're fun. I think you chase after things. But I think you're frightened you actually might fall in love with a girl. So you don't let anyone get close.'

What a nerve. I cursed the person who hired her, then realised that person was me.

'Rubbish,' I said, 'that's such bull—'

'Is it?' she said, walking back into the building. 'Is it really?'

And uncharacteristically, I couldn't even attempt a witty comeback.

Close to five in the morning the Portuguese woman arrived in a taxi. It was one of those ordinary saloon cars. They're white and green in Brighton. Before it had even come to a stop, the door flung open and she came charging towards us. In one arm she carried a cat carrier, in the other a plastic bag. She was short with thick dark hair, and hazel eyes. Instead of using the bell, she rapped on the front door with her knuckles until Ruth came running to her assistance. She introduced herself as Mrs Lopez before pushing the carrier towards me.

'Is mother in the basket, Mr Abraham,' she said. 'Is egg in the bag, Mr Abraham.'

I peeked into the cat carrier, the mother hissed. She was a beautiful tortoiseshell queen. She was lying on her stomach, not on her side, and she didn't appear to be in labour, she looked exhausted. I looked at the new mother then back to her cat-sitter. Mrs Lopez thrust a carrier bag under my nose, but kept hold of the handles.

'It was in the wardrobe,' she said.

She opened the bag so I could see inside.

'I open bedroom door and find this in wardrobe, Mr Abraham.'

I stared down into the white plastic carrier bag at the greenish placenta at the very bottom.

'Mrs Lopez, did you see any kittens in the wardrobe?'

She looked at me and shook her head. 'It is full of clothes and boots, Mr Abraham.'

I put my hand on her shoulder. 'I think we better take a proper look.'

It was our first home visit. We piled out of the trusty new red Cinquecento onto the pavement outside her house. The lady lived in a block of flats not far from the practice. It was one of those unattractive blocks from the 70s, named something like *Sandringham* or *Weston*. As we walked towards the front door, I noticed a large blue sign that read NO DOGS ALLOWED EXCEPT THOSE BELONGING TO RESIDENTS, next to PLEASE KEEP OFF THE GRASS, and another which read NO BALL GAMES followed by NO FOULING. Four in a row, what party poopers the council are. She lived on the top floor and the lift wasn't working so we hurried up the stairs – I counted 79 – Mrs Lopez leading the way with her cat carrier, me behind, and Ruth bringing up the rear with the carrier bag.

'This is the bedroom,' she said, flinging open the door. It was a small chintzy room containing a big pine double bed with a white duvet and floral throw, a pink side table with hundreds of photos in differently sized frames, a pine dresser against the wall and a huge pine wardrobe.

'Sssh!' said Ruth. 'Do you hear that?'

Mrs Lopez set down the cat carrier and knelt on the floor.

'*Eeeeeee!*' went the wardrobe.

Mrs Lopez's eyes came out on stalks.

'*Eeeeee!*' it went again.

I didn't move. Neither did Ruth, as Mrs Lopez crawled on hands and knees across the garish pink rug towards the wardrobe. She stopped and looked around.

'Open it,' I whispered.

Mrs Lopez reached forward and touched the corner of the door with her fingers. She picked at the under-side and gently pulled it towards herself.

'*Eeeeee*!' It was more than one voice.

We all crept forward to have a look in. Very carefully Mrs Lopez swept aside some of the dresses that were hanging on the rack. The kittens' cries grew louder. And standing a couple of feet behind, we watched Mrs Lopez crumble as right at the back of the wardrobe was the most precious of things, a litter of five baby kittens.

That sight could warm the hardest of hearts. Ruth and I spent half an hour with Mrs Lopez and the kittens. We told her what she had to watch out for, and showed her how to care for them. It was best to leave them where they were for now and reunite them with their mum. Mrs Lopez said she was going to call one of the fattest ones Marc and the thin one Ruth. I wasn't sure whether to be flattered or offended.

We were soon back in the car. After Ruth's unfair comments about my car earlier in the evening it had taken surprisingly little persuasion to get her into it. I mean, I had given it a fairly good sell. Conscious that words like 'clever' and 'practical' could come back to bite me I sold it on the premise that is was 'fun', like a go-kart. I will agree that to many car-owners obsessed with leather and litres, walnut dashes and grunt, our tiny Cinquecento may have seemed laughable, but it would get us from A to B (though maybe not to C). Now I am by no means a small man but I could sit reasonably comfortably in the front, so long as the seat was pushed back. We waved goodbye to Mrs Lopez and headed back to the practice. Sadly for Mum's sleep tip advisor, I couldn't find a Christian rock station, but I tuned our radio in to Classic Rock. The stereo danced along to the soft eighties beat of 'Purple Rain'. Ruth and I looked at each other and without provocation we launched into our own Karaoke versions, mine with a Red Bull microphone, hers with a deodorant can. We sung all eight minutes and forty seconds of it. And when it ended Ruth looked out of the passenger side window, and I looked dead ahead, as if the whole thing was completely premeditated.

Two roads away from the surgery, Ruth piped, 'So why don't you have a girlfriend?'

I pretended she wasn't asking me again.

'Well, I don't care what you say,' she said, 'I'm gonna make it my mission to find you one.'

And she grinned from ear to ear.

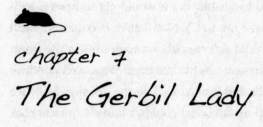

chapter 7
The Gerbil Lady

Let me tell you about the day I became Brighton's first and foremost gerbilologist, if such a thing exists.

The practice had been up and running for a couple of months when I took the call. As a vet you meet a lot of characters, and Fleur was something of a local celebrity. An ardent Brighton and Hove Albion fan, she would regularly turn up to the practice on a windswept Tuesday night in a replica shirt and scarf with a patient to drop off before the match. She was my most regular client. This had something to do with the fact that she kept well over a hundred gerbils. Which, obviously, was how she came to be known to us as the 'Gerbil Lady'.

On the day I was to establish my gerbil credentials, Ruth and I pulled up outside her house in our sweet red Cinquecento. The practice phone had been diverted to Ruth's mobile and we had Blu-tacked a laminated notice to the front door – *Back in a little while*. Ruth had insisted on drawing a picture of a 'see you later' alligator underneath it. Fleur lived in the very last house of a quiet residential road. From the front it looked like any normal, suburban house, but if you were able to see a satellite image of the property the first thing you'd notice would be the large black extension stretching out of the back of the house and two large sheds, which served as aviaries.

Fleur's husband, Roger, ran an animal rescue centre. 'Ran' is maybe too soft a word for it. This was not a nine-to-five job, Roger devoted his entire life to the care and rescue of animals. From rehabilitating seagull chicks that had blown off townhouse roofs, and pigeons attacked by the peregrine falcons of Sussex Heights – a famous block of flats in town overlooking the West Pier – to unlucky fledglings snatched by worried owners from their cat's jaws. Roger and Fleur's house was not so much a home as a sanctuary for wild animals. Their garage was like one of those huge stuffed bird displays at the Natural History Museum but with a hundred heart-beats and various whistles, chirps and pips, that got louder with every approaching tweezer of cat food. People would drop by with seagulls and swifts, but also hedgehogs and badgers and fox cubs and strays, and would think nothing of ringing their doorbell at ten o' clock, midnight, and two in the morning. It was incon-venient at times but Fleur and Roger wouldn't have it any other way.

We parked behind their little blue car in the drive. They had a large Seagulls sticker on the rear window:

the emblem of the football club and a bird that was more than a recurring theme in their lives. Ruth and I stood outside the front door rubbing our hands together to keep them warm. The South Coast was in the grip of a cold snap that the weatherman blamed on a 'sudden arctic pocket', whatever that was supposed to mean. It's funny how many fancy words and phrases they have to camouflage the truth that they never saw it coming.

'Hello, Marc,' said Fleur, and she leant in for a hug. Our breath made vapour trails in the air.

Fleur was a wonderful woman. Short, huggy, and warm like a radiator. She was bursting with a passion and love for life though nothing could quite top her love for gerbilkind. Fleur was more than a breeder, she was a gerbil evangelist, with a website dedicated to their upkeep, and her own gerbil version of the Ten Commandments, which she laminated and gave to every new owner. When she opened the door we were greeted by a newborn curled in the palm of her hand. It made embracing a little tricky. I went for a sort of side-hug.

'Come in, come in,' she said, 'the kettle's boiled, I'll just be a second. Tea?'

'Thank you,' I said.

Ruth was a few steps behind me. When she saw the baby gerbil face peeking out of Fleur's hand, she melted into a mushy puddle, and let out a cutesy 'awwwwwww' before asking for a 'stwoke'.

We warmed our hands and toes by the gas fire as Fleur steeped the tea. Ruth looked wistfully towards the kitchen and made coochy-coo faces. Their house was an Aladdin's cave of animal affection. There were paintings and photographs in every conceivable place, clocks, ornaments and cuddly toys. There were gerbil plates, gerbil mugs, gerbil draught excluders.

Ruth perched on the edge of the sofa cushion as if we were visiting the house of an eccentric great-aunt, and couldn't quite relax. Fleur chinked and clinked away in the kitchen, but over and above it you could hear the sound of animal industry – the pitter-patter of five hundred tiny feet. Ruth's eyes flicked from one corner of the room to the other as she tried to work out where it was coming from. I nodded towards the pair of interconnecting doors. The dining room was something else. Ruth had never been in the house before, but I'd warned her about the dining room on the drive over.

'The sound alone,' I told her, 'is like nothing you've ever heard.'

For all the animal goings on, the household had a restful air. It's something that you often find with people who are doing what they were put on this earth to do. Fleur and Roger had one of those star-crossed stories. They had met on a late-night show for BBC Southern Counties Radio, where Roger had been a guest presenter. They still produce a radio show every month called

Roger's World and record it in their home studio. Roger presents while Fleur operates the controls and chips in every now and then. They make a wonderful team, and they've been doing it long enough for each to know what the other wants without so much as a word passing between them.

Fleur pushed herself up on the balls of her toes and looked out of the living-room window as she came back with mugs of steaming tea.

'I'm sorry you had to make the trip out in this,' she said, looking out into the frost. 'Roger had a call from a lady about a badger and had to use the van, so I couldn't come over myself.'

Ruth was hoping a little face might be peeking out of a fold or a pocket in her sweater, but Fleur must have put the baby gerbil somewhere else. She set our mugs down on the coffee table on World Wildlife Fund coasters.

'That was when I noticed something was wrong,' she said. 'I'm sorry, what am I doing? Let's take them through.'

Fleur picked the mugs back up off the coasters and pushed them into our hands.

'You're okay carrying them, aren't you? We're in here. Marc, you've been here before, haven't you?'

I took a little slurp.

The dining room was separated from the living room by two white sliding doors with frosted glass panels.

With a little tug, Fleur pulled them open and I watched Ruth's face light up like a Christmas tree.

They still called it the dining room though it had long stopped playing that role. Three of the four walls served as apartment blocks for gerbils. They were like four star high-rise gerbil hotels. Gerbils are social creatures so Fleur had divided them into breeding pairs and allocated their own love nests, complete with water bottles, twin beds and exercise equipment. There were 154 of them in total. Each cage was labelled with their names – which usually began with an S – painted on to a nameplate, which was cut into the shape of a rainbow and hung underneath the cage. Their cages themselves were decorated with clip-art that had been simply cut and pasted from the Internet. These gerbils lived in luxury. I'm sure Fleur would have wired in little telephones and mini-bars if the gerbils could use them. Every day each pair was allocated a few minutes to stretch their legs and run on a purposely built gerbil gym while their love nests were given a thorough clean-out and inspected for new arrivals.

The sight of the accommodation itself was a spectacle to behold, but it was the sound that really hit you. Gerbils are not noisy animals but with 154 all talking, playing, drinking, squeaking, and running round their wheels at once, the sound was other-worldly, like we were trespassing amongst the Lilliputians. Ruth hurried straight over to the cages, and was going along like a child in a pet shop.

'You'll have to excuse her,' I said. 'I wasn't aware that she had such a thing for gerbils.'

'No,' said Fleur, 'it's quite understandable.'

'I wuv their wittle fwaces,' said Ruth, pushing her own up to the cage.

Fleur was beaming. 'Do you keep gerbils?' she said.

'When I was growing up,' said Ruth, moving on to the next cage.

I felt bad about separating the furry rock stars from their latest adoring fan, but there was a pressing matter to attend to. One of Fleur's gerbils was in a protracted labour. Shirley had been having contractions for over 24 hours without delivering. A gerbil usually rests for 15 minutes between deliveries to conserve energy, but a wait of this duration was a sure sign something was seriously wrong.

'I'm assuming there isn't a chance of saving the babies,' said Fleur.

Shirley was lying on the straw at the bottom of a tank. Her teeth were chattering in pain. I looked up at Fleur, concern written all over her face.

'And she's been like this for a day?' I said.

'Almost two,' Fleur replied quietly.

'Okay,' I said, pausing, 'Fleur, I have to warn you, but after two days I don't think – I mean I might be wrong – but I think it's unlikely this will be good news for the babies.'

'I thought so,' said Fleur, 'that's fine. I just want Shirley to be alright.'

'The thing is, Fleur,' I said, 'she might not be alright, if the babies are stuck inside.'

I looked into Fleur's eyes. They were strong and stubborn.

'That's why you're here,' she said. She paused, stretched out her hand and gently squeezed my arm. 'I've done my research and I know it's really super uncommon, and most vets wouldn't touch this, and I understand why, but I'd love if you could perform a Caesarean.'

I gulped. 'A Caesarean?'

I wanted to make sure I had heard her correctly. In the veterinary world it's almost unheard of to hear the words 'gerbil' and 'Caesarean' in the same sentence, let alone be asked to perform one.

I looked from Shirley to Fleur and from Fleur to Shirley and a lump the size of a gobstopper grew in the back of my throat. Though I had never done anything like it, or, for that matter, heard of such a surgery being performed, there was no way I could stand in her home and refuse her, and before I even knew what was happening I heard these words leaving my mouth, 'Ruth, could you fetch my bag from the car?'

Fleur's big eyes welled up with tears.

*

As much as I would have liked it, my bag was not one of those old leather doctor's bags that the medics in *Poirot* carry, it was a large plastic box with tiers of shelves inside, like a fisherman or an electrician might carry. There are a great many tools to carry on a home visit. Usually we would have some idea what case we were about to see and pack accordingly, but Fleur had been reluctant to explain the nature of the problem over the phone for reasons that were now painfully obvious.

Ruth took Fleur to the living room to sign the consent forms, while I racked my brains to try to remember what they had taught me at vet school. I don't know if there was ever a lecture in small animal Caesareans, but if there had been I must have been off that day. I looked at the gerbil sitting next to my hand. Shirley was no more than six inches long, including her tail that made up almost half the length. The incision I was going to make would be absolutely minute. If you've ever made an Airfix model plane, you'll appreciate what I mean when I say it was fiddly. I searched around in my bag for the smallest, thinnest scalpel blade I could find, and placed it on the top of the table. The other trouble was anaesthetising her. Small animals are usually put under by placing them inside a container and introducing gas into it. Normally I'd use a plastic box in the practice to make a small chamber, but because we didn't know what we were coming to, we hadn't brought one with us.

'Fleur,' I asked, 'do you by any chance have a clean margarine tub?'

'Hmm,' she said, 'I don't know.'

'I need a tub of sorts, to anaesthetise her.'

'Hang on,' she said, 'I'll be right back.'

Fleur nipped off to the kitchen. I looked at Ruth through the gap in the connecting doors, kneeling by the coffee table, and I looked at the scalpel blade, and I looked around at the Gerbil tower blocks and began to regret saying 'I'll do it,' with quite the bravado I did. I mean, where do you start? It was my Superman complex kicking in. Riding in like a knight in shining scrubs on my big white stallion. Maybe I was being too hard on myself. This was about Fleur and Shirley, and I knew that if I didn't operate Shirley would die, so there really was no other option.

'Ice cream anyone?' said Fleur, swinging into the living room with a newly washed out tub. 'Raspberry Ripple,' she said, 'I've scooped it into a bowl if you fancy some after.'

This wasn't the time to start contemplating dessert. I looked down at Shirley on the table and back up to Fleur again.

'Look,' I said, 'I want you to know that I'll give it my best shot, but I've never done anything like this before...'

'Don't worry,' said Fleur, 'I wouldn't have called you if I didn't think she'd be in the best possible hands.'

We put the pregnant gerbil under in the ice-cream tub that served as an anaesthetising chamber, and as Fleur stroked Shirley's soft fur with the tip of her finger, I clipped carefully around the gerbil's abdomen. We were all three crowded around the side table in the dining room. Ruth had cleared the space, and scrubbed the surface clean before laying down a plastic sheet. We were dressed head to toe in aprons and masks, and I insisted that we each wore a pair of sterile rubber gloves. And, as we three giant human beings leant over the tiny sleeping gerbil, I reached for the scalpel, and with the smallest blade made a minute incision, as 153 gerbils watched on. Sadly, all three of the baby gerbils never made it into the world alive. By the looks of things they'd been dead for over 24 hours, and were shrivelled like peanuts in their shells. Fleur wiped a tear with her sleeve and both Ruth and I battled to remain unaffected. I spayed Shirley when she was asleep and set her on course for an uneventful and speedy recovery. When she was stitched back up, Fleur threw her arms around me and clung so tight I didn't think she was ever going to let go.

Somehow the whole incident affected me on a deeper level than I had imagined. Ruth and I didn't talk much on the journey home. It was a kind of euphoria mixed with a sense of mission, if that isn't too strong a word. Most of the time you do things that you see day in day out, and they become a routine, but there are times when you are invited to reach for something above and beyond, and it's those times that you remember why you're there.

We were driving back to the practice when Ruth noticed that she had a voicemail. She wasn't much of a techie, so it took her a little while to get to her answerphone.

'Press one,' I said.

She growled at me.

'Two new messages,' she said, repeating the automated voice.

It was drizzling again, and the wipers were making a squeaking sound on the windscreen. I watched Ruth's face out of the corner of my eye as I focused on the road.

'Korma meal? Mild set meal,' she huffed, shaking her head.

'Two poppadoms?' she tutted.

'One. King. Prawn.'

Her voice rose.

'NO!' she yelled into the phone. 'You cannot have a free pilau!'

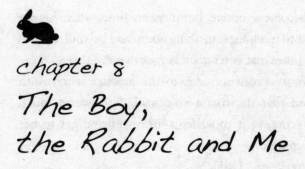

chapter 8
The Boy, the Rabbit and Me

In the weeks since Ruth threatened to find me a girl-friend I became aware of a conspiracy against me. It seemed that the female-to-male ratio of owners at the surgery, which had been about 50–50 at my old practice, was now it was close to 70–30. Not that I was making tallies in my notebook, but this was how it seemed to me. Of course, the logical side of my brain told me it was purely coincidental, but in the part of my mind that's home to my paranoid gland, there was a creeping suspicion that my nurse was playing Cupid. Ruth did, after all, regulate who came in to the surgery and who didn't. She was in sole charge of the telephones. And, it wouldn't have surprised me if it wasn't herbal teas she was brewing in the kitchen, but love potions. Thankfully so far she hadn't tried to set me up with any of my clients, though I had a feeling that was about to change.

It was a Thursday night and the surgery was relatively quiet; a few things that could be dealt with over the phone, one or two drop-ins, but nothing like the mad rush on the weekend. We saw a dog that had been involved in a fight and a five-month-old German shepherd who'd been vomiting for five days.

I was in reasonably good spirits, but hadn't had much sleep on account of a friend's birthday lunch. I turned up at one of those family pubs on about three hours' sleep and stumbled my way through a steak and Guinness pie, in between slurps of lime and soda. Matt worked freelance and had the afternoon free to set up base-camp in a corner of the bar, so that his other friends could drop in during their lunch breaks. Being a night-worker, I was the only one who didn't have an office to go back to, so the responsibility of keeping him company as he drank his way through his birthday pints fell squarely at my feet.

The lack of sleep meant I arrived at the practice with a grump on my face. I think Gloria took one look at me, opened her mouth, as if to say something sharp, then just as quickly shut it again. She was adept at reading situations. In fact, the next thing I knew there was a cream bun on a plate by my bag. I think she took pleasure in mothering me.

I was relieved that the evening wasn't too demanding. The dogfight was as bad as it got. It wasn't so much a fight as an attack. The victim was a Staffie, who had been out on a walk minding her own business, when she was set upon by a Lab cross. Clearly no one had told her that bull terriers were meant to be the tough ones. It wasn't until her owner pulled the other dog off her that the damage stopped. He had carried her, bloodied and injured the half a mile home and then brought her in to us. She had bite wounds on her leg, neck and ears and pretty serious swelling.

Some people ask me whether distressed animals affect me or whether seeing it day-in, day-out deadens the emotional impact. The short answer is that no matter how many times it happens, seeing animals in pain is upsetting but you can't let it get in the way of doing your job. And there's no better feeling than bumping into a dog walking with its owner that you saved from a road traffic accident three weeks before.

I administered injectable antibiotics to keep the bite wounds from becoming infected. I looked at her, lying there, covered in battle-wounds. It's usually Staffies that are cast as the aggressors. As I got to work with suture material and an ice compress, it served as a strong reminder against those that stereotype breeds.

Lucy, a German shepherd, was up next. She hadn't been responding to the medication she'd been prescribed by her own vets to control her vomiting. I pulled up the skin at the back of her neck to make a tent shape and it was very slow in springing back. She was chronically dehydrated, passing diarrhoea and sleeping for most of the day.

There's a lot that could be wrong, so she'd need a full-on clinical investigation. The emergency surgery remit was, as the name suggests, to treat emergencies and prepare them for their regular vets to do anything that could wait until the following day. So we made sure she was comfortable and kept her overnight with an intravenous drip, to be thoroughly checked over in the morning.

I was walking back from the inpatients overnight ward when Sally, a full-time single mum, walked in to reception with her eight-year-old son Harry, who was clutching a large cardboard box. I'd been to Harry's school a couple of times to talk to the children about National Pet Week or Bonfire Night. I love school visits, especially when I take in a special guest; a dog, a mouse, or a snake. The children's eyes go wide like saucers. My favourite part is the question time at the end, you never know quite what topics you'll end up fielding. At the last school I went to we spent over 20 minutes talking about the proper funeral arrangements for fish. When one kid brought up his fish story it was like he had fired a starting pistol, all the others started chiming in – me, me, me. The boy with the ginger hair told me how his black fish ate his blue fish, the girl with braids mentioned how she forgot to feed the fish when she went on holiday and they were all floating on the top of the tank when they got back, and then the tubby boy in the corner told the class that his uncle has a shotgun. I don't know how much they really take in, but when I walk back to our practice afterwards, I picture them excitedly telling their parents in the car home from school what they'd learned and scuttling out into the garden as soon as they get in to check under their bonfires for hedgehogs.

Sally and Harry turned up at half past ten with their rabbit, Emily, wrapped in a warm blanket, inside a cardboard box. Harry was wearing his red and blue Spiderman pyjamas, a green stripy bathrobe and slippers. His teeth were brushed, he was ready for bed, but the pained, worried look on his face said that something serious had happened. Sally explained the situation to me.

Harry loved playing with Emily and Emily loved to run around the living room, so when Harry came home from school, the first thing he'd do after he'd set his schoolbag down at the bottom of the stairs, was go outside to her hutch, scoop her in his arms and carry her in while Sally got the dinner ready. Emily was a French Lop rabbit. She was a plump little thing with short little legs. She had these beautiful long floppy ears that hung down with the tips below her jaw. Her fur was a beautiful sooty fawn colour. French Lop rabbits are quite big, so they can be challenging as house rabbits, you need to let them have plenty of space.

Harry would settle down on a beanbag to watch television while Emily bounded and hopped around the living room. Harry made her obstacle courses. He put overturned cardboard boxes, cushions and pillows on the carpet, and carefully placed a line of carrot batons from the start to the finish to mark the route. Harry found it hilarious to watch her hop around the carpet and would score her as if he was judge for a TV dance competition. Unlike Bruno Tonioli, however, he spent most of his time trying to fish the competitor out from under the sofa and get her back onto the course. Emily would sit on his lap while he had dinner, and Harry would feed her the vegetables he didn't want. And before Harry went up to the land of nod, he'd carry Emily back to her hutch and say goodnight.

But that evening when Harry walked back into the living room, Emily was lying unconscious on the floor. Next to her was a frayed lamp cord and her mouth still around the wire.

A cardboard box with a mop of floppy hair and two red Spiderman legs walked into the consulting room. Harry insisted on carrying it with the flaps up so he could see inside. His eyes were streaming with tears. Sally guided him in with a hand across his back and helped him settle the box on the table. It was the first time Harry tipped his head up. He looked up at me and his eyes filled with tears and emptied on his cheeks.

'Don't worry,' I said.

'I'm so sorry,' he said to me, as if I was a rabbit too.

'It's not your fault,' I said, 'this happens all the time.'

He wiped away the tears with the sleeve of his pyjama top. As I lifted Emily out of the box and studied her frazzled face, I looked into Harry's and I saw myself in his shoes, a little boy standing exactly where he was, in a veterinary surgery in Stanmore, North West London.

'When I was your age,' I said, squatting down to his level, 'I had a tabby cat called Suzy. Boy, did we get up to some mischief.'

I put Emily down on the table.

'Really?' he said.

'Lots of trouble, yes,' I said.

'Like what?' said Harry.

'I can't tell you with your mum here,' I whispered.

Harry grinned from ear-to-ear.

'Go on,' he said.

'Another time,' I said.

The truth was we did get into trouble.

There is one event in particular that is forever seared into my memory. Suzy was an elderly mackerel tabby with a coat of dark browns, ochres and black, and beautiful curvy stripes. We were like Darwin and Captain Fitzroy, trekking off to unknown corners of the garden, capturing never-seen-before creatures and displaying our haul on the kitchen table, as it were an expo at Kew Gardens.

We'd hang out in the garden as often as we could. I used to draw all the animals in my sketchbook. Suzy thought I was wasting my time. At first she'd purr and claw my jeans, make pleading, playful whines, then she'd curl in a ball at my feet, and go to sleep. I had a thing for butterflies and over the course of a half-term Suzy-cat and I became expert netters. The best time was early mornings when my family and the butterflies were in their roosts. Suzy would wait for me at the bottom of the stairs with an expectant paw on the bottom step, I'd be in my striped pyjamas. We'd tiptoe into the kitchen and make sugar-water juice in a plastic jug. I'd sprinkle it on the buddleia and baste it on to the backs of my hands in the hope of teasing one over to feed through its long proboscis. The trick was to creep up from behind like a careful Elmer Fudd. Sudden movement startled them into flight and there's nothing more frustrating than going one footstep too far, muslin net above your head, to see the target flutter away as if you'd tripped a laser beam.

One particular Sunday afternoon I was in my camp as usual. It was the end of half-term. The garden was filled with spring and I was wearing my Arsenal away top – yellow and blue, before they went green in the 80s. We'd been there twenty minutes when a chocolaty thing floated by on the breeze and landed on the buddleia. It took me a few seconds to realise what it was, but when I did I went stiff like a statue.

'Watch the Admiral,' I whispered to Suzy. She eyed me from her daisy patch and made a puzzled frown. 'Keep your eye on him,' I said.

The equipment was on the patio. I could make it there and back in about 40 seconds if I walked out fast and crept back slow. My arms were raised and my elbows were up to my ears as I held the net ready behind me. Every muscle in my face strained in careful concentration. Suzy-cat slunk down onto the lawn as I inched towards the buddleia bush. The Red Admiral was sitting pretty, lifting and lowering his wings like he was making little breaths. The net bag made a swishing sound as it whisked through the air in front of me and out the other side.

'Ha-ha,' I sang, 'I got you,' and I swept the net forward and flipped the bag over. The Red Admiral didn't fly out. The Red Admiral was never in. As I boggled at the empty net, I saw him fluttering higher and stop at the top of the fence. He beat his wings if as he was laughing at me, which I didn't appreciate much.

'Come on then, you toad!' I shouted, wagging my fist. 'Come back and get what's coming.'

Without thinking I scooped up a stone, and screwing up one eye for aim, launched it as hard as I could at the butterfly by the fence, the fence that bordered the neighbours' house, the neighbours' house with the brand-new greenhouse, the brand-new greenhouse that made an ear-shattering sound as the stone sailed into a pane of glass and sent shards splintering everywhere. I stood rooted to the spot. I didn't dare move a muscle. I waited for an angry shout, a gunshot or a curse.

Nothing.

My first instinct was to slowly turn my head to make sure I hadn't been spotted. The second was to climb the neighbours' fence and retrieve the evidence. The fence was twice as high as me and made of thick wooden panels. There were no handy holes to reach for or nails for my feet but if I clambered on the stump of the rose tree I could lock my fingers over the top. With a push up I could see over. But I hadn't figured out what I was going to do when I got that far. I heaved myself up with my arms so my chin rested on top but my shoes were swimming in the air. I tried to grip them on the fence, but I couldn't get any traction. They scrabbled desperately, my chin slipped back towards me, and then my arms gave up. I came crashing to the earth and my Arsenal top snagged on the hawthorn tree. I knew I shouldn't cry but it had been signed by Liam Brady and when I finally yanked it free the sleeve was completely torn. And as I wiped a tear away the Red Admiral fluttered by.

It was hours before the neighbours found out. I watched their car pull into their drive from the chair by the living-room window. And when the neighbour stomped across our front lawn with a face as chocolaty-red as the butterfly, there was only one thing for it. I hid under my bed and made a hedge of dirty laundry. Oh, to be eight years old again. Like Harry.

I felt a tug on my scrubs.

Harry was smiling at me.

'Let's take a look at her,' I said.

While I checked his rabbit's eyes, Harry scuttled around the table to get a better look. Emily normally scrabbled around in the box and wrestled with the vet. So when Harry saw her, still and quiet, he pursed his lips.

'Don't worry, Harry,' I said, 'she'll be fine. She's had quite a shock, that's all. Does she play in the living room a lot?'

Harry looked at his mum, then back at me and nodded his head. Usually when advising clients to 'proof' their houses it's regarding a new puppy or kitten; naturally curious fluffy youngsters who can easily land themselves in trouble if not adequately protected. But with this country's recent and continuing huge increase in owners choosing house-rabbits over dogs and cats, I find I'm giving the 'rabbit-proofing speech' more and more – especially on the run-up to Christmas – when fairy lights can be potentially lethal.

'Suzy-cat and I used to play all around the house like you and Emily,' I said. 'You just need to be extra careful with rabbits because they'll nibble just about anything. Their favourite thing is wires. Emily can play in the living room, you just have to make sure the wires are hidden

away, or thread the wires through some plastic tubing –
you can get that from a hardware store.'

Harry hung off every word I said. His floppy brown
mop swivelled round, atop his hazel eyes. He looked at
his mum. She nodded.

'He wants to be a vet when he grows up,' said Sally,
ruffling his hair. She threw me another smile.

'Well, you can help me then,' I said. 'Do you want
to come round here?'

The corner of Harry's mouth picked up and he shuffled towards me. I asked Harry to hold Emily's rear end
while I opened up her mouth.

'Good job,' I said.

Ruth passed me a torch.

'We use this to have a good look around,' I said,
'there we go.'

I didn't take long to locate the affected area.

'Ruth, can you take over from Harry? I think I'm
going to need his opinion on this one.'

Harry walked round to where I was standing.

'Hold the torch,' I said. 'Now have a look in while
I keep her mouth open.'

Harry gripped the torch and shone it around his
rabbit's mouth like he was investigating a sea cave.

'Can you see in there?' I said.

Harry nodded.

'What can you see?'

He shook has head.

'Can you see that she's burned her tongue?'

He screwed his eyes up and looked at it. He wrinkled his brow.

'She hasn't,' he said.

'She has,' I replied.

'Why isn't it black, then,' asked Harry, 'if it's burnt?'

Sally laughed. 'It's not a piece of toast, Harry,' she said.

Harry looked up at us and then began to laugh. He tipped back his head and laughed and laughed. Which got us all going. I winked at Sally. Then Harry suddenly stopped laughing and looked at me.

'Is it bad?' he said.

'It's not great,' I replied. 'She'll be in pain for a bit, but it'll heal. I'll give her an antibiotic and a painkiller now to make her feel better.'

'Like Panadol?' he asked.

'A bit like that,' I said, 'but in bunny-sized quantities.'

Harry smiled as he pictured what that would look like.

'I've got a joke,' said Harry.

'Go on.'

'Why are there no painkillers in the jungle?'

'I don't know, Harry,' I said.

'Because the parrots eat them all. Get it?' he said.

'No,' I said, because I genuinely didn't.

'Parrots-eat-em-all, silly,' he said.

'Very good,' I said. 'Now, Harry, we need to talk about feeding. Burns can take several weeks to heal. And if a rabbit doesn't want to eat, she won't eat.'

Harry's eyes went wide again, as he took every word in.

'Try her on her food as soon as possible,' I said, 'but she may not take any. If she doesn't, then you may need to syringe feed her.'

'I don't have a syringe,' said Harry.

'I can give you one,' I said, 'Ruth, will you fetch a fairly big syringe for Harry?'

'I don't like needles,' said Harry.

'Oh, there's no needles,' I said.

'Then how do I inject her?' said Harry.

Sally chuckled. 'We're not injecting her, Harry,' she explained. 'We'll feed her food. In her mouth.'

Harry thought we were joking. 'Squirt it?' he said.

'That's right,' I said. 'Get some baby food, or liquidise some vegetables, and feed her a small amount with a syringe.'

Harry nodded. 'Did you remember that?' he said to Sally.

Sally smiled. 'Yes, Harry,' she said. 'Let's not take up any more of Mr Abraham's time. Thank you so much for helping us.'

She held out her hand.

'No trouble at all,' I said, shaking it. 'Come and see us again.'

I knew Ruth was watching me, but I wasn't going to look in her direction. I picked Emily off the consulting room table and put her back in her box.

'And thank you, Harry, for helping me out,' I said, as he held out his arms and I passed him the box.

'Now, Harry, if we get busy with animals and I need some help, is it okay if I call you?'

Harry looked at me over the cardboard box and his eyes went huge.

'Really?' he said, 'You serious. Do I get my own outfit?'

'Of course,' I said.

'Then yes,' he replied. A great big smile twisted from one ear to the other. I wished them both a safe trip home and led the way out to the car park. I stood by the window and watched Harry buckle the cardboard box into the back seat and lift the flaps to check Emily was okay. He turned back and waved to me as they pulled out into the road, and they were gone. I opened my mouth and let out an almighty yawn. How much longer was there to go?

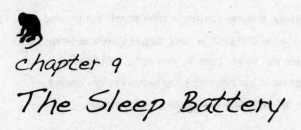

chapter 9
The Sleep Battery

From: Mum
Date: Thursday, 17 March, 9:43 pm
Subject: This Might Help You

Marc,

Your father found this on the Internet. Maybe you
should check it out but make sure it has been
properly tested.

RSVP
Mum x

SLEEPACELL – The Sleep Battery
How many times have you gone out for a night out
and crashed? Or been working late and just plain
run out of steam? Now imagine a world in which you
could sleep when you have time to and be wide
awake when you don't? It's time to put those
yawnful days behind you. SLEEPACELL is a sleep

battery. It works just like a solar panel, but instead of storing energy on a sunny day, it stores up sleep when you've got time on your hands. If there's nothing in the diary flick the battery on to 'charge me up' and bank a few hours for a busy day.

How it works. Attach the electrodes pads to either side of your temple and relax. Caution: Do not use with water beds.

THE SLEEP BATTERY

From: Marc
Date: Friday, 17 March, 7:32 am
Subject: Re: This Might Help You

Mum,

How are things? Thank you for your email. As I
mentioned on the phone, I'm doing fine now, I've
really adjusted well to the hours.

I Googled SLEEPACELL the sleep battery and could
only find one mention of it on a weird website. It
looks great but I think I'll wait until it's picked up
by a high-street retailer before I hand over control
of my brain.

Marc x

PS: What was Dad doing on a site called Monkey
Juice?

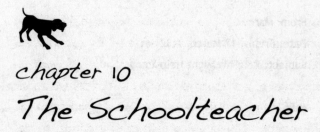

chapter 10
The Schoolteacher

When I arrived at work, there was an envelope waiting for me. It was a big floppy homemade envelope, made from a piece of blue foolscap that looked as if it had been torn from a scrapbook. It was stapled rather haphazardly at the edges. My name was scrawled across the front in fairly childish writing, along with a rather surprisingly accurate picture of my smiling shaven head, here drawn bald. Each letter of my name was written in a different coloured pen. I sat and admired it for a few minutes, not wanting to rip it when I tore it open. Ruth was in the kitchen whisking herself up an Echinacea drink and adding things that looked like twigs from a Tupperware box. 'Don't ask,' she'd said as I walked in.

'I got a card,' I said, waving it under her nose.

'Oh yeah,' she said.

'Hand-made,' I said, knowing girls are impressed by hand-made things.

Ruth had a long-handled teaspoon in her glass. The sort you might use for a knicker-bocker glory to get the strawberries out of the bottom. She stirred it clockwise.

Stopped. Turned it anti-clockwise. I opened the kitchen drawer and pulled out a teaspoon of my own. It was regular-sized, as teaspoons should be. I needed an implement to get under the staples. Ruth watched as one by one I unpicked the envelope and flapped open the folded paper. Inside was a picture of a rabbit. In the bottom right-hand corner in crayon it read: 'Dear Marc, thank you for fixing Emily. When I grow up I want to be like you. Lots of love Harry.' And after his name he had written 'Aged 8¼' for which he earned bonus cute kid points. I put it on my desk, next to the *Little Britain* DVD that had come in the mail.

I've mentioned how I try to not become too emotionally drawn in to some of the distressing situations with patients, but it is impossible to be completely detached. It's often not the patients themselves but the owners who can create the biggest pressures.

We were having one of those nights. The waiting room was full. I'd finish treating one case and walked back to greet the next owner to find three more patients waiting. One of the stresses with Emergency Surgery is having to prioritise clients when we're busy. Emergency shifts are weird. You can be sitting around for hours, punctuated only by the occasional phone-call or ward-round, but it's usually when you're busy dealing with an emergency that another one is on the way. And when they just turn up at the clinic, it can be the real test; to prioritise, or 'triage', and get the best outcome for both or more cases that are presenting at exactly the same time. It's stressful at times, but can be such an adrenaline rush, and with time you're able to teach yourself subconsciously how to achieve an even calmer state the busier and crazier it gets. It can be a real test of people skills too, because it's not only the poor animals that we're treating here. Every pet owner naturally considers their emergency to be more important than anyone else's, but as an emergency vet when lives are at stake you often have to let a frustrated and anxious owner know that you have to see to another animal first.

I was standing in the waiting room, trying to assess which of the three patients needed to be seen next, when we had a walk-in road traffic accident. A dog had been 'scraped' off the road – knocked down minutes earlier and scooped up into the arms of a concerned animal-loving motorist or passer-by. Hit-and-runs don't just happen with human beings, the main difference is that the chances of someone stopping for a dog on the side of the road are remote.

It was a white Jack Russell cross, about three years old, wrapped up warm in the nice stranger's fleece top that she didn't mind getting blood-stained. The stranger deserved a medal. She was in her late forties. She told me that she'd just popped out to get some gravy granules from the shop for her toad-in-the-hole when she saw the hit-and-run, and now here she was in the practice offering to pay for the animal's treatment, even though for strays it's always free unless an owner eventually does come forward.

Ruth scanned the dog around its shoulder area for a microchip, but no joy. I don't want to get on my soapbox, but microchipping is the frontline in reuniting pets with their owners, there's no sane reason not to do it. The scanners pick up a unique code that can locate their owner within a matter of minutes. In road traffic accident cases, there's no chip more often than not. The situation is often made worse by the collar and nametag having been ripped off in the accident too.

We checked over the poor dog for a tattoo, but there was no way of identifying him. He had cuts and grazes to his head, clustered around his eyes where the skin is thinner over the bony arches of the skull. His left ear was torn and bleeding. He also had a suspected broken left foreleg at the carpus, which I'd already noticed, flapping around as he was brought into the clinic. Ruth estimated his weight, and I drew up some quick-acting pain relief, injecting him in the thick thigh-muscle of his back right leg. He was pain-free within a few minutes. Some road accidents need to go straight onto oxygen, some are dead on arrival, so in the wide spectrum of outcomes ours was a lucky one, so far, at least.

Ruth took the details from the lady who was kind enough to stop for him, where he was found and what she had seen. I could see the lady was thinking about things. Some people bring in an animal they find, and, knowing that it is in safe hands, are happy to disappear. This lady wasn't like that; she wanted to stay around, to make sure he was okay. She was there when we administered painkillers, she watched as we cleaned him up, and when there was nothing else to see, she still hung around, just to make sure. Just before she left, the lady reached into her purse and pulled out a scrap of paper. She picked up a pen from the counter and with a shaky hand she jotted down her phone number and handed it to Ruth.

'If he lives, and no one comes forward,' she said, 'I'd like to take him on.'

Ruth and I stopped what we were doing.

'I've decided I'd like to take care of him,' she said again.

'Really?' Ruth said. 'That's amazing. Amazing. Thank you.'

She leant forward and gave the lady a hug.

'Have a think as to what you would call him,' she said.

'The obvious one would be Lucky,' she said, 'or what about Mr Bump?'

Ruth smiled.

'You better get back to your toad-in-the-hole,' I said. 'We'll call you and let you know how he's doing.'

*

Whenever I'm having a low moment, I play back scenes like that one. I can still see the look of intensity in the woman's eyes as she pulled out the scrap of paper. It's amazing how such a significant thing can be expressed in such a simple action like that, and how it totally restores your faith in the human race; if, that is, you overlook the day a similar scenario occurred only for the 'strangers' who brought the dog in turn out to be the owners, but they didn't actually admit it. They were after the free treatment. It's hard not to be cynical sometimes.

Lucky, or Mr Bump, or whatever his name was to be, really was lucky to have that lady walking by. He was still shivering so we put him on a heat-pad, warmed-up a bag of saline, and inserted a drip into his right foreleg. The dog wasn't castrated; he was probably knocked down chasing a bitch in season, which would have made it a totally preventable accident. I gave him some antibi-otics and some more pain relief intravenously and made him comfy in his kennel until he was stable enough to be sedated for x-ray. You can never be sure if they'll let you but we attempted a pressure bandage on his ear, and Ruth gently bathed his wounds and scrapes, then went back in the direction of the waiting room. I peeled off my gloves and threw them in the waste bin. It was like in a Hollywood movie, when the lead looks over to his co-star and says something like 'Don't call me a hero, I'm just doing my job.' I think it's okay to feel proud of what you do once in a while.

I looked over to the wall clock, sucked in a deep breath, and breathed it out again. It was not even ten o'clock.

'Marc, there's a lady who needs to speak with you,' said Ruth.

I shut my eyes for a moment, and rubbed my fingers over them.

'Right,' I said, 'give me a few minutes.'

'I think you should speak with her.'

'Well, tell her I'm just wrapping something up,' I said.

'She's not here. She's on the phone.'

'Ruth,' I said, 'I'll call her right back.'

'Hello?' I said, with a note of trepidation.

I perched my bum on the desk, I didn't even have time to pull up a seat. Ruth had been lingering outside the consulting room door, so that as soon as I had walked out, she intercepted and rushed me over to the office. What on earth was the matter? She scooted me down the corridor with her hand across my back. Steady on. The phone was lying on the desk. My only thought was that the caller must be agitated or threatening, or something. But she was neither of these.

'Marc,' she said, 'lovely to hear your voice. It's Fern.'

I hate it when they just tell you their first names. My

head was doing somersaults trying to pin a face. I know several Ferns.

'From the primary school,' she added.

'Miss Gilmore,' I said.

'That's right,' she said, 'but call me Fern.'

'I'd better call you Miss Gilmore,' I said, 'otherwise I'll call you the wrong thing in front of the kids.'

She laughed. Then there was a pause. A clunky one, like you get when you don't know who should speak next.

'Is everything okay?' I said.

I looked up at the door to catch a glimpse of Ruth's uniform disappearing as she sailed off down the corridor.

'Well, I wanted to call about my cat, but first I wanted to thank you for helping Harry's rabbit,' she said.

I took a second to process what she was saying.

'Harry's rabbit,' I said, baffled. 'You mean Emily?'

'Yes,' she said, 'the class couldn't believe it when Harry said you'd brought her back from the dead.'

'Well, I wouldn't go as far as to say that. Children will exaggerate, Miss Gilmore,' I replied, 'as I'm sure you know too well.'

'Yes, well, Harry said she'd been electrocuted and her heart stopped, and you got it going again.'

'It wasn't quite that dramatic.'

'But still, Marc, it was so great of you to take such care. Emily is pretty much the class pet. We're not allowed to keep one at school, but Harry volunteered to bring her in. We're studying *Watership Down* in English.'

'Right,' I said. 'Well…it was nothing.'

'I'm sorry,' she said, 'this must be embarrassing for you.'

I beckoned Ruth with my finger as she walked past the door again. She threw a quick smile and carried on.

'Er… Miss Gilmore, is everything okay? I mean, was there something you wanted to talk to me about?'

'Oh yes,' she said, 'Marlow's eye is gummy.'

'Marlow is your…?'

'Cat,' she said, 'he's a Burmese. I found him cowering behind the sofa, in full daylight. And then I noticed his left eye was watery, today it's bright red, and all gummed up. I mean, I thought twice about phoning because I wasn't sure it was an emergency as such and I didn't want to make a nuisance.'

I scratched my head.

'You know your animal better than anyone else, Miss Gilmore. If you're worried about your pet, you should never feel embarrassed. Why don't you pop down straight away and I'll take a look at him?'

'Are you sure?' she asked.

'Of course, bring him down, sounds like conjunctivitis, so I'll take a good look.'

She thanked me and said goodbye and I put the receiver down. I put it down on the desk and stared at it for a minute. What was that about? The marching me down the corridor? There were other patients waiting. I turned around to see Ruth make another unscheduled walk past the door.

'Ruth…' I said.

'No time to talk,' she replied briskly, 'we've got a lot to get through.'

'But why…?'

'Marc,' she said, raising her voice to such a level that everybody in the practice could hear, 'there are patients in the waiting room. Can we have this conversation when you've seen to them?'

There's a part of me that has always wondered whether I should be a teacher. You can imagine what a joy it would be to look out every day at thirty eight-year-olds and nine-year-olds. To sit behind a desk or walk amongst them, and talk about things that happen in their worlds. Maybe it's a slightly romanticised perspective. I bet at times they're a right pain.

Miss Gilmore had been teaching at the primary school for five years. Everything about her was soft. From her curly brown hair, to her chunky knot cardigan, to her toilet-tissue-soft voice. As an eight-year-old I imagine she could still appear terrifying, but only because she was a teacher.

That evening, as she walked in the door, I noticed that she had a bashful way about her. She sat her cat carrier down and smiled at me. It was a primary school teacher's smile – big, white and sunny. A smile that sings 'The Wheels on the Bus', a smile that tells the children to put their coats on when they go outside, and that counts their heads to make sure no one is missing. She reminded me almost exactly of my teacher at school, when I was Harry's age – Miss Jennings.

Miss Jennings was a little bit older perhaps, and not quite so slim, but she had that same smile. I think when I went to school the teachers were stricter, and didn't try to be friends with the children, but Miss Jennings had a soft spot for me. She loved animals too, so we'd often talk about local wildlife, and she was always keen to see the sketches that I did in the garden. We got on well, apart from the, er, bat incident. Yes. The bat incident. Crumbs.

I remember sitting in her office, staring at the tiles, and swinging my legs under the chair, as my mother read her the riot act on letting children take things home from the nature table. The 'bat' incident that incurred my mother's wrath happened the day before I returned to school from half-term. I can still see my sister Danielle screaming in the kitchen. And Mum up on a kitchen chair with a rolled-up *Sunday Times*. Danielle was hiding under the table, screaming scarlet into her face, as the thing swooped down and dive-bombed the lino floor. It wasn't a bat at all, but a Poplar Hawk Moth. I remember telling them calmly but it was as if I was speaking Greek. It wasn't a problem. I fetched my butterfly net from the dining room and as the moth made another swoop I swung it in front of me and bagged him in the muslin. Danielle went silent. Mum's arms froze in a mid-air.

'It's a Poplar Hawk Moth,' I said again, holding it though the net, 'they're totally utterly harmless.'

Then Mum clambered down from the kitchen chair and dragged me off to the hall. She pointed down at my school bag.

'What was it doing in here?' she said.

'Was what?'

'The moth,' she said.

I made a not wholly unconvincing shrug, pretending not to know about it.

'I asked Danielle to get your school bag ready, Marc, and that wretched thing flew out.'

'He was a chrysalis when I put him in,' I said, 'he must have hatched out in half-term.'

Mum's eyes went big and white, and her face filled up with red, from the bottom to the top. I had taken the chrysalis from the nature table at school. It was just one of those things that boys do.

*

Miss Gilmore stood over the consulting room table.

'Has it been busy?' she said.

'It's been a long old night,' I said, 'and it's not even halfway through.

'And you're sure I'm not taking up someone else's slot?'

'Please, Miss Gilmore, we don't have "slots".'

She bent down to open the cat carrier. There was a soft meow from inside. Miss Gilmore reached into the cat carrier with both hands and lifted him onto the table. Marlow was a beautiful cat. I have a soft spot for the Burmese breed – strong, elegant, athletic. You just want to sit in their presence and dote on them like royalty, set down a velvet cushion. Marlow had an exquisite soft blue-grey coat with a silver sheen. He was like a miniature panther. He was muscular and heavy to lift. It's funny to watch someone who's not used to the breed try to pick them up, the weight of them always catches people out. I have friend who calls them 'bricks wrapped in silk'.

'Hello, Marlow,' I said, hoisting him up.

Marlow showed signs of swelling of his left eyelid and conjunctiva. His left eye was weeping and almost fully closed with pain, though his right eye didn't seem to have any problems at all. If it had been the same in both I would have guessed he'd had some contact with an irritant, or perhaps an allergic reaction.

'I'm sorry about this...' said Miss Gilmore, looking at the time.

'About what?' I said. 'Eye health is very serious. Would you like a cup of tea, Fern?'

'No thanks,' she said, and a smile broke out on her face.

'Will you hold his backside?' I asked.

'Of course,' she said.

Burmese can have a predisposition to glaucoma, and I was anxious to discount that possibility. I needed to examine the eye but you want to make sure it was as painless as possible, so I gently teased back his eyelids and squeezed in a local anaesthetic eye-drop. Waited a few seconds then got out my torch. He squinted and pulled his head away, but I managed to see everything I needed. There was too much discharge for glaucoma, and it wasn't just watery, but gunky and yellow. His left eyelid was crusty.

'Looks like conjunctivitis,' I said. 'It could be that a tiny foreign body got in – like dirt or sand or hair and it's become infected.'

Marlow was in discomfort and the cause of his conjunctivitis was still a mystery. Top of the list would seem to be a scratch or an ulcer on the cornea. Given that Marlow had only been like this for a couple of hours a scratch seemed most likely, either from a scuffle with another cat, a head-on collision with a sharp twig in the garden undergrowth or in pursuit of one of the birds in the hedges. The next step was to assess any corneal damage. I took a damp orange dye-soaked strip of paper and touched it on his eyeball. Any scratch will usually bind to the dye and turn it green – which you can easily see with an ultra-violet light when the room's dark. I flicked off the light. There was a definite green cloud shining from the seven o'clock position. With the lights back on, gently pulling back the lower eyelid revealed the tip of a grass seed that had snuck its way in and was rubbing on Marlow's eye, and it was made worse with every blink. I left Marlow and Miss Gilmore while I went to find some forceps. It was an easy task to remove the seed now we knew where it was. I got out some antibiotic eye-drops.

'I'll show you how to put them in, and then see if you can do it three or four times a day.'

Miss Gilmore was very attentive and listened to everything I said. I handed her the eye-drops.

'You may as well use this one,' I said. They were already opened, so it saved her the cost.

'Thank you.'

We put Marlow back in his carrier, and small-talked for a few minutes. Miss Gilmore went to leave the treatment room, when she stopped, and turned back around. I noticed she had stopped out of the corner of my eye, but continued to update the computer records.

'Marc?' she said.

She looked down at her toes then she looked back up again. I looked over, and came out from the desk.

'It's really nothing,' she said, 'I mean, I know you're extremely busy. It's just I wondered if you ever used work-experience kids?'

I smiled.

'Forgive me for saying,' I said, 'but aren't you a little old for that?'

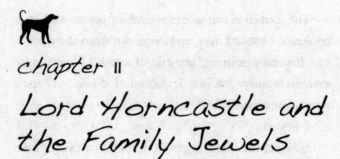

chapter 11
Lord Horncastle and the Family Jewels

Lord Horncastle was one of those people who looks defeat in the face and carries on regardless. This may have a little to do with his family motto '*Invictum est fatum*' or 'fate is invincible'. If you were to spend any length of time with him at all you would realise that one area he was not lacking was self-belief. Lord Horncastle was a vocal man and liked to have his say on local issues. He saw this as his responsibility. And whilst you would rarely see him on the front page of the newspaper you only had to turn a couple to find him caught in some controversy about footpaths or by-laws, or extolling the virtues of organic farming, something he knew little about but felt he ought to, what with him being a lord, and gentry and all.

Lord Horncastle was exceedingly tall. He was at least a head taller than every other member of his family, and would joke that his parents' milkman was an ex-NBA basketball player. Lord Horncastle did not however possess the athleticism of a basketball player. He was skinny and awkward and never out of suits and wellies. I had met him once before. We were both guests at a special Remembrance Day Service in Hyde Park, at the Animals In War memorial, which was well attended with animal-lovers wearing purple poppies. Lord Horncastle was lined up for a reading about a donkey and I gave a speech about the welfare of animals in current war zones. After the service was over, I rode back to Sussex with him and his wife in their Land Rover. I held onto the head rests and spent the entire journey leaning forward like a little boy who didn't want to be missing out on anything. Lady Horncastle was an animal rights campaigner, which was quite unusual for a member of the gentry. She had all sorts of stories about the times her views put her at odds with a lot of her peers, many of whom were still battling the hunting laws. It bore testimony to a strong impulsive streak that I can certainly relate to. My favourite story was about a recent dinner party that they held. Lady Horncastle was so outraged that a lady had arrived wearing a fur hat that she had it taken from the cloakroom and burned it in front of them as they ate their vegetarian quiches. We talked about all sorts of things, but mostly about animals. I heard all about the animals on the family estate, which would have given Noah and his ark a run for his money. Lord Horncastle was fairly matter of fact, rolling them off like an inventory, and Lady Horncastle would chip in with names and fill me in on the fluffier details, comparing them amongst each other like they were cards in a game of animal top trumps. They had horses, sheep, goats, cats and chickens, not to mention all the wild animals they fed. But the reason our paths would cross at the emergency practice was to do with a darling of the family – one of Lord Horncastle's dogs.

Horncastle had always bred German shepherds.

'If you could cross a human with a German shepherd, I daresay they'd be a lot of smarter than we are. Even if you just spawned enough to be teachers, we could sort out this country's education system in a jiffy.'

I didn't know how to respond.

'Imagine a *University Challenge* team facing those half-breeds. They wouldn't stand a chance. Muscular, agile, very loyal. Every football team should have one,' he said. He looked at me with a smug grin and slapped me on the back.

'Have you ever had a German shepherd?' he asked.

'No,' I said.

'Do you have children?' he said

'No,' I replied.

'Good for you. If I could turn back the clock, I would have had less children and more Germans. Come outside and have a look at this one.'

It was just past nine o'clock in the evening when Lord Horncastle's Land Rover pulled into the car park. The car was splashed in mud. So much so that it looked like it had been through a car wash where the water had been swapped with chocolate milkshake. In the back of the car was the silhouette and striking pointy ears of a German shepherd. Ruth looked out from the window, sipping a caffeine-free acai berry tea, as Lord Horncastle regaled me with another one of his tales. I stood back as he opened the boot. It was one of those beautiful balmy spring evenings that presage what would hopefully be an awesome summer – not that I would get to see much of it.

'What's his name?' I said.

'Ferdinand the Second,' he said, 'after the King of Prussia, not the Holy Roman Emperor.'

He was a fine specimen of a German shepherd, about six months old, and immaculately groomed. Lord Horncastle took him by the collar and led him off onto the ground.

'He's in fine shape, Lord Horncastle,' I said, giving Ferdinand a cursory look over, 'what a beautiful dog. So, what's up?'

Lord Horncastle coughed twice, and adjusted his jacket in a rather theatrical manner, then in a hushed tone he bent over and in a quiet, low tone said, 'It's not so much what's up as what isn't down.'

He pulled himself back up and stroked his chin with his finger, like a university professor poring over a riddle.

'I'm sorry,' I said, 'I think I'm missing something.'

Lord Horncastle gestured downwards with his finger, pointing towards the ground.

'Do you want to explain?' I said.

'No testicles,' he whispered, presumably so Ferdinand would be spared the blushes. 'No family jewels.'

I had a look at Ferdinand's underside.

'He's six months old, Mr Abraham, I thought they'd have dropped by now, and we're showing him in three weeks' time. I've had a look at finding them, it's like looking for misplaced car keys. The boy's been giving me some strange old looks,' he said.

Lord Horncastle was obviously very proud of his dog.

'Look at him,' he said, walking round to face Ferdinand. 'Noble head, keen expression. Eyes set obliquely and not protruding. Ears pointed in proportion to the skull. Arched forehead, look how perfect that is. The skull slopes beautifully into the muzzle. Jet black nose. Wonderful strong jaw. Good teeth. Muscular neck. Straight back. Capacious chest. Well-sprung ribs. Bushy tail that curves like a sabre. He a prize-winner. An absolute cert... and then we get down here and it's, wait a second, where's the giblets?'

He was boasting, but not without cause. Ferdinand was a magnificent dog.

'Well?' said Lord Horncastle. 'Where are they?'

We went inside and I laid him down on the consulting room table. Lord Horncastle paced around the room, as I made my examination.

'What?' said Lord Horncastle. 'What have you found?'

'The ring hasn't closed.'

He stopped pacing.

'What does that mean, old chap?' he said.

'It means he could be a late descender.'

I felt around his lower abdomen.

'You can normally feel if something's wrong. What I mean is there's still time for them to drop. Some dogs take twelve months or so. The trouble is,' I said, 'I can't feel them. Do you want to try?'

Lord Horncastle reached in and put his hands where mine had been. I showed him where I was pressing.

'Cryptorchidism,' I said, 'giving it its formal name, is a fairly common condition although usually just on one side not both. It can be relatively straightforward to fix if the un-descended testicle can be palpated externally, but more often than not, as in this case, it can't, which means it's somewhere between his kidney and bladder area. I'll be honest, after this amount of time, the odds aren't in your favour. But we should just keep monitoring it.'

Lord Horncastle looked at me.

'There's a chance they will never drop, and if that's the case, eventually you'll have to get him neutered. But I think there's a good chance they will.'

His look turned into a glower.

'Did I say the wrong thing?' I said.

'The show's in three weeks' time,' he spluttered, 'how can we speed things up?'

'If we could locate them then we could try to massage them into place, but there really isn't any way of "speeding it up", as you say.'

'Can't you operate?' he said.

'I know it sounds easy to sort out but the operation to fix and remove the un-descended testicles can be quite tricky and lengthy as they're usually tiny. There's no simple way to find them, the X-rays won't usually show them up and they are typically very small. The operation can take some time. You have to make a long incision and once you're inside you begin the search by going to the kidney and working backwards, follow-ing the testicle's chronological path of development to the scrotum.'

'Pah. But you must be able to do something,' he harrumphed.

'Just get your vet to monitor it, and if they don't

drop you'll have to have him neutered. An un-descended testicle can become cancerous, and it may produce more testosterone because it's at a higher temperature.'

Lord Horncastle couldn't bring himself to look at me. He made dark eyes at the floor.

'Would you give him implants?' he suggested.

'Absolutely not,' I said.

'We'd only do it temporarily, until the others descended,' he said.

'Try to massage them into place. We need to give him a little longer and monitor things. I have a good feeling they'll descend,' I said.

'How much to...?' he said.

I looked him straight in the eyes.

'Lord Horncastle, I wouldn't do it.'

He glowered at me.

'Come on, boy.'

And with that he led Ferdinand by the collar out of the consulting room, got into his car and drove away muttering his family motto under his breath.

I walked back along the corridor, turning it over in my head. I was right to say what I said, there was no way I would give the dog implants, certainly not until we'd seen if the others could descend.

Ruth was in the office watching the *Little Britain* DVD for the umpteenth time, curled up in an easy chair, tipping her head back and roaring with laughter, though roaring would be the wrong word for it, when she laughs she honks like a goose.

'You're never going to believe what I've just been asked,' I said.

Ruth was totally absorbed in the DVD.

'Marc,' she said, pointing at the telly, 'did you see that?'

Honk. I hadn't but there was no way I could stop myself from laughing along with her. I don't care who you are, honks are contagious.

'You're never going to believe what I've just been asked,' I said again.

Ruth stopped, pulled herself up in her chair like she'd had a revelation, and turned to look at me. 'Oh,' she said, 'I haven't told you, have I?'

'Told me what?'

She got up out of her seat, pushed past me in the doorway and raced off to the kitchen. She came back clutching a shiny yellow flyer in her hand.

'There,' she said, 'read this!'

She shoved the flyer into my hands. It was a cheap, badly designed thing that folded into three.

'New Sundarban Bangladeshi Takeaway,' I said. 'I'm more a Chinese man myself,' I said, handing it back.

'No, stupid, look at the phone number.'

My eyes darted down to the phone number printed across the bottom and up to our phone number printed on the laminated sign above the desk. I got to the last three digits and stopped.

'That's our number,' I said.

She nodded. The penny dropped.

'Oh,' I said. 'No way.'

'Yes way.'

'Hence all the orders for curry?' I said.

'Exactly,' said Ruth with a smug look on her face that would have given Poirot a run for his money.

'Did you ring them?' I asked.

'Yes, they were ever so grateful. They asked if we could give out their correct number, switch the seven and the three?'

'We're not directory enquiries, Ruth.'

'I know, but they said we could have a free order of anything on pages one and two.'

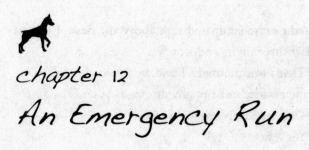

chapter 12
An Emergency Run

Gloria was waiting when I turned up, in her sweet Welsh way. She was wearing a big red sweatshirt and these crazy parrot earrings, swinging in gold hoops. Gloria always had a different song to greet us with when we turned up for work. It was either a schmaltzy number from a bygone era, a Max Bygraves or Perry Como, or a kitsch disco classic, usually something by Donna Summer. As soon as she caught sight of me walking across the tarmac she broke into a stage school version of 'The sun has got his hat on, hip hip hip hooray' and even before my trainers had reached the welcome mat, she took me by the hand and asked for a dance. I have always fancied myself as a James Bond-type character; and Gloria was the closest thing I had to Miss Moneypenny. I took her in my arms and we waltzed a couple of laps around the waiting room. I hasten to add that I didn't join in with the singing, that would have burst the bubble. She giggled as we spun around the coffee table, stacked with issues of *Country Living* and *Sussex Life*.

'Any messages for me, Miss Moneypenny?' I said with a wink.

'Two,' said Gloria, beaming and she twirled. 'One from a lady who says she has decided on a name, let me see if I can remember. I think it was one of the Mr Men...'

'Mr Bump?'

'That's right,' she said, and she laughed to herself. 'I thought it was a sweet name. Mr Bump, yes, Mr Bump and she can come and collect him this weekend.'

'That's great,' I said. 'She was the road traffic accident lady. The one I was telling you about.'

Over the past few days he had made a startling recovery from his orthopedic surgery. We'd still need to keep him in for a few more days, but it was great that the lady was still as keen as mustard. They were going to be good together. We danced another lap of the coffee table.

'That's right,' she said, 'now what was the other call... oh yes, a teacher called Fern. She asked if you'd call back.'

Miss Gilmore wasn't after work experience for herself, she was asking on behalf of her sixteen-year-old nephew Dan, about to start college, and very interested in a career as a vet.

'I told him he can come for a day trial with you, and if things go well, well... I didn't promise anything,' said Miss Gilmore, coyly, 'but I might have said that if things go well he could stay a bit longer, perhaps.'

I looked up at the calendar pinned to the wall. We only used it for dates and marking in holidays, gigs and comedy nights, there were never any work entries. One of the bonuses of the emergency shift is that you don't have to be adept at forward planning.

'That's fine,' I said. 'He's not squeamish, is he? It's just that we do see some pretty gory things from time to time.'

'Oh, I wouldn't worry about that, he loves *Casualty*,' she said.

I laughed.

'Look, I'll call him and fix a time for him to come in for a talk next week, and if he's keen then we could get him started when term ends.'

'Perfect,' said Miss Gilmore. 'Now when are you going to see my class again, they've got hundreds of questions?'

'Sometime soon, send me over some dates,' I said. 'How's Marlow getting on?'

'Oh, how rude of me. He's *so* much better. His eye's a tiny bit pink, but the gunk's gone and he's so much happier.'

We said our goodbyes and I put the receiver down.

'How was Fern?' asked Ruth, with a smirk.

'If you are referring to Miss Gilmore,' I said, 'she's fine.'

Ruth and I hadn't talked about Fern. Ever since Fern had come in with Marlow, Ruth had waltzed around the practice with a minxy grin on her face. So whenever Miss Gilmore's name came up I changed the subject immediately.

'What sort of night are we going to have tonight, do you reckon?'

'I just hope it's not a quiet one,' said Ruth, 'I'm not ready to start the *Friends* box set over again.'

On reflection 'I hope it's not a quiet one' was a foolish thing to say. It was one of those lines you catch coming out of your mouth, that usually precedes an evening from the pit of hell. In fact if you played the scene back, I bet you could hear the snidey tone of the voice-over man saying something like, 'Be careful what you wish for.' I didn't see any television cameras, but it was one of those surreal evenings where you expected Jeremy Beadle to pop out from behind a bush and tell you it was a great big wind-up.

Cecilia is one of those names that isn't very common nowadays. Simon and Garfunkel should bear the responsibility for this; no right-thinking parent would name their daughter after a girl whose sole claim to fame was afternoon love-making. I happen to think Cecilia is a sweet name, and when it popped up on my computer screen, I smiled. Then the biggest dog I think I have ever seen came into the consulting room.

Cecilia was an Irish wolfhound with the stature of a

small pony, in fact. Had I been naming her, I would have started with something like 'Jumbo'. She was grey and her coat was shaggy and wiry, and she had a fantastic bushiness around her eyes, like they were hiding behind Brillo pads. She was muscular and strong, and had she been able to stand up straight on her hind legs, she would easily have dwarfed me and Mike, her owner.

Mike was a furniture salesman and an amateur football referee on the weekends. He was tall and athletic. He and Cecilia lived in a two-storey townhouse. Working in an urban practice, you don't see many Irish wolfhounds; they need a lot of exercise so are more commonly rural pets, but Mike and Cecilia were both keen runners, and when Mike finished work every day he'd would change into his running vest and tracksuit and take her out for a five-mile run, as anyone who has ever visited the Withdean Sports Complex between the hours of six and seven can testify. She'd run alongside him for a while then tear off on her own, race another dog, come back and run alongside for a bit and so on.

Today was pretty much like every other weekday. Mike finished his last sales call and returned home. Because it was a Friday, he left his car at the local garage for its annual service. One of the mechanics gave him a lift home, and Cecilia was, as ever, waiting at the bottom of the stairs for him to come through the door. She left him a couple of minutes to hang up his jacket and take off his shoes before shuffling over to ask how his day was with that 'about time' look on her face. Mike had his banana, got changed and the pair left the house for the walk to the sports complex.

Irish wolfhounds' lifespan can vary between four and ten years. Because of their size, the temptation is to take them out running too young. Their overstretched limbs can cause irreparable damage. But when they're Cecilia's age, they can give Linford Christie a run for his money. Cecilia was three years old and she absolutely loved to run. Mike walked her to the park then as they came around the final bend he'd let her off the lead. Cecilia was an obedient dog, and knew to wait until they were on the grass before sprinting off. She waited while Mike did his stretches, and warmed himself up.

At first, Cecilia appeared fine. When they were in the house, Mike noticed that she hadn't eaten much, but he thought nothing of it at the time. But the minute they left the house there were signs that something was wrong. A mile or so up the road, she began to wheeze. At first Mike thought she must have eaten something strange, that it would pass as she swallowed, but when he finally let her off the leash she just stood there with her head and neck extended. Cecilia was having terrible trouble breathing.

*

Cecilia's neck was extended so that her head was held straight out and made a straight line with her back. She was drawing breaths like she was having an asthma attack, her chest was caving and it sounded like she was gasping for air. They had come straight to us on the way back from the park; Mike still had his water bottle in his hand. He set it down on the table. He was wearing his Adidas tracksuit, and there were beads of sweat on his forehead from exercise and nerves, which was perfectly understandable. As soon as I saw her, I knew it was serious.

'Has she ever done this before?' I asked.

'No,' he said. 'It came on really sudden, two hours ago she was fine.'

My first thought was that it was pneumonia or even heart failure. It can be especially difficult with Irish wolfhounds because it comes on so quickly. One minute they're fine and the next they're definitely not.

'Has she had a cough?' I asked.

'No, she's been fit as a fiddle,' said Mike, 'seriously, seriously, healthy, no problems.'

I leant in close to her chest. Another common cause is something getting stuck in the lungs. Her chest wall was pumping like a pair of bellows.

'Mike,' I said, 'I don't want to alarm you…'

'Okay,' said Mike, nodding.

'If she has any of these conditions, we're going to need to see to it right away.'

'What does that mean?' he said.

'Well first I want to X-ray her to make sure there's nothing obstructing her airways, but...'

'But what?' said Mike.

I got out my stethoscope and knelt down beside Cecilia so I could listen to her lungs. The sound of healthy lungs is clear, what I was hearing was crackles, like the sound of Velcro, a sign there was fluid in the lungs.

I raised my head and looked at him. With a normal-sized dog an X-ray is never a problem, but with a dog that weighs more than most adult human beings it's too big for our clinic's X-ray table.

Ruth passed me my coat and shoes. Mike was already waiting with Cecilia by the Cinquecento. He had his hands around his eyes like binoculars, pressed up to the glass so that he peered in through the windows.

'We won't fit her in,' he said. 'I should run back and get my car. Oh wait, it's in the garage.'

'We'll be fine,' I said, 'the hospital's not far.'

I don't say this too often, but in moments of crisis, Ruth is a complete genius. She had walked into the consulting room to check up on us, to find Mike leaning with both arms on the Formica desktop, desperately trying to hold it together, while I racked my brains to think of some way we could X-ray Cecilia. The problem was the equipment we had was designed for animals much smaller than an Irish wolfhound.

'Maybe we could try it anyway,' I'd said.

'It won't work,' said Ruth.

So I asked Ruth to get on the phone and try to find us a facility for larger animals. Ruth sprinted down the corridor to reception and started leafing through Gloria's address books. She tried another animal hospital just a little out of town, but their machine was the same as ours. She phoned the university, but couldn't find anyone that was still around. There was one place in Brighton with a facility large enough. It probably wasn't used to requests like ours, but there was nothing to lose. So, with her best telephone voice, Ruth made the call, then came running into the treatment room.

'We're in,' she said, 'if we hurry.'

Ruth, herself was out of breath now.

'In where?' I asked.

'Brighton General,' she said panting.

'Brighton what?' I said.

'General.'

'The hospital?' asked Mike.

'Yes,' she said. 'I called the switchboard and was told that the duty radiologist would call me back after being bleeped. Which he did, and luckily he loves dogs, too.'

We were all crowded around the car.

'There's no way we'll fit all of us in,' said Mike.

'It's not far, we can all squeeze in,' said Ruth. 'Help me with the back seats.'

We opened the boot and set to work, pushing the buttons on the tops of the seats to push them flat, and clearing the junk out of the boot. I hoped Mike wouldn't spot the rust hole. We laid a blanket down to make things more comfortable for Cecilia; I wasn't sure we were going to get her to lie, she was still standing with her neck extended to help her breathe. With stroking and calming words we managed to coax her into the boot and with a little encouragement she lay down.

'You okay?' I asked Mike.

He nodded.

'Buckle up,' I said. 'It really isn't far.'

'It's only half a mile up the road,' said Ruth. 'They know you're coming.'

Mike buckled himself into the passenger seat and I skirted round to the driver's door. There wasn't enough room for Ruth, and I wanted Mike to be there. When Ruth closed the boot it acted like a sound box, the wheezing was amplified. I reached for my seat belt, and put the key in the ignition, turning it to the right to start the engine. But nothing happened. I turned the key back and tried again. Nothing. I could see out of the side window that Ruth was already halfway back to the practice. I looked at Mike and made a nervous smile, pulled the keys right out, shook them, and inserted the key again. Paused for a second then turned it firmly to the right. Still nothing.

'Oh no,' said Mike, staring straight ahead.

'I'm not sure what's happening,' I said.

I looked up at the rear-view mirror and saw Cecilia staring back.

'What now?' said Mike.

'We'll get there,' I said.

Inside, I shrugged my shoulders. The air firing in and out of Cecilia's lungs was harsh and wheezy. Suddenly there was a loud knock to my right; I turned to see Ruth's knuckles rapping on the side window. She opened the door.

'It won't start?' she said.

I didn't have to answer.

'Don't worry,' she said, 'it's not far. Let's use that.'

She pointed over by the wall.

My eyes travelled to where she was pointing. I looked over the wall, and beyond, expecting to see a taxi, or something, anything. But there was nothing.

'What?' I said.

'There,' she said.

'What?' I said.

'The shopping trolley,' she said. 'Come on. It's only half a mile.'

She ran over to the wall, grabbed the abandoned trolley by the bar and dragged it over to us. I laid a piece of hardboard over the top of the trolley while Ruth nipped inside to get some more blankets for cushioning. That was the easy bit. How do you lift an Irish wolfhound? Cecilia weighed over a hundred kilograms. We opened the boot and reached in. Mike put his hands under her stomach and forelegs and I supported her rear end. It took several minutes and a lot of repositioning before we were able to lift her enough for Ruth to get her hands under her middle. The crackling sound of the air fired in and out of her lungs. The poor dog was fighting for breath. Somehow we managed to get her onto the trolley, and laid a couple of thick grey blankets on top, so she was covered from her chin to her feet. We had her positioned so that her head was at the end that I was pushing. Ruth volunteered to take the front of the trolley and Mike ran alongside talking Cecilia through it. We came out of the car park, and turned right, flying down the street.

I could never have foreseen how much her weight would inhibit the motion of the trolley. The trolley was so over-loaded, it handled like a galleon. They're not the easiest things to steer at the best of times so you had to make sure you were setting off in the direction you wanted to go, you couldn't manoeuvre it if you tried. Thank God it didn't have a wonky wheel. It took both me and Mike leaning our full weight and pushing hard to get the thing going; God knows how we were going to stop it. Thankfully the roads were clear. We were tearing along the road like a bobsleigh team. Ruth guided the front with her hand locked round the basket, yelling to anyone in her path to get out of the way. They stepped aside as we clattered by, with the sound of racing wheels on tarmac and shuddering metal.

Brighton General Hospital is a huge late-Georgian building that was built as a workhouse and infirmary in the nineteenth century. The principal building is an impressive four-storey edifice, with large windows, four gables, a clock tower and these stone dolphin decorations. As we clattered round the final bend of the road the clock tower came into view, with its domed lead cap that looks like a pepper pot. The car park was ludicrously busy when we got there, as you would expect for Friday night. We weaved in between cars and pedestrians. The tarmac had an incline and we hadn't gathered quite enough speed to keep the momentum going, so Mike dropped to the back to help me push, tugging the left-hand side of the trolley to steer us out of the way of a BMW. As we wheeled Cecilia down the drive we passed a pair of students supporting a limping drunk friend, with blood streaming from his head like a war casualty.

'Cover her face,' I shouted to Ruth, as we slowed our sprint down on approach. Ruth took the ear of the top blanket and pulled it over Cecilia's head, allowing her a little space to breathe. We came to rest at the entrance.

'Where now?' said Mike.

'Stay here,' said Ruth, 'I'll run in and sort every-thing out.'

We pulled up outside the electric doors, and Ruth ran up to the counter. The waiting room was packed. There were mums with sons with bandaged heads, old men in wheelchairs, smart women, scruffy drunks, all of them clutching a tiny slip of coloured paper with a black number printed on it, indicating their place in line. A mother filed out with her son's arm in a plaster. The son looked at Mike, and me. Then stopped. He whispered something to his mother. She turned and stared, then hurried him on. Cecilia's tail was hanging out.

Ruth came charging out of the doors.

'Okay, we can go straight through now,' she said.

'Where?' I said.

'In there,' she replied, pointing to where she'd just come from.

'With a shopping trolley?!'

Waiting for us in the ambulance bay was a proper hospital trolley with two porters. It took all four of us to transfer poor Cecilia from our makeshift wheels and whisk her straight through A&E, past the semi-conscious drunks and insomniacs, and into the radiology depart-ment where she was X-rayed. We were done and back at the clinic within the hour, clutching fantastic black-and-white films of her lungs. It brought the confirmation we needed that there was no foreign body in her lungs or dangerously enlarged heart. We kept Cecilia overnight on an intravenous drip and started her on a course of antibiotics. Within three weeks she was fighting fit again, tearing around like she always did, and waiting at the foot of the stairs for Mike to come home for his run. It would have made a very nice ending if I could have said that I'd bumped into Mike and Cecilia while I myself was out running in the park, but I'm afraid to say, I'm no runner.

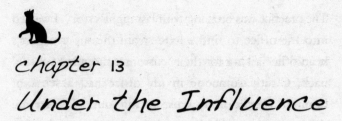

chapter 13
Under the Influence

'Heavy night, Marc?' said Gloria when I arrived for work for next day.

I look at her a little disappointedly.

'It took me a long time to get to sleep this morning. Do I look bad?'

'Oh no, you never look bad, Marc. But you do have a large red-wine stain down the front of your hoodie. It looks more like a slick than a spill.'

I looked down at my zip-up hoodie that I had grabbed before I left the house.

'It's urban camouflage,' I said. 'Don't worry; I have had a shower. Smell me if you don't believe me.'

I don't know how I could have missed the stain. The thing was, I had fallen asleep in front of the television, and woke with wine soaked into my clothes, and the sofa. The menu screen of *24* was on the TV with a thirty-second music clip looping. It's never the best way to wake up.

'You need a woman in your life,' said Gloria.

'Not you as well,' I said.

*

The practice was buzzing with last night's story. I walked into the office to find a letter from the supermarket's head office asking for their 'customer shopping vehicle' back. Clearly someone in my office had a sense of humour. A schoolboy sense of humour. Now let me think who that could be.

'Above and beyond, that was, Marc,' said George on his way out. 'Were you after some bonus Nectar points?'

He laughed and made a gun with his hands like schoolboys like to do in the playground.

'Well I hope you have a less adventurous night tonight, try to keep your James Bond instincts to a minimum,' he said. 'Don't you think, Miss Moneypenny?'

'I do,' said a beaming Gloria, 'unless of course he wants to take me out in an Aston Martin, and then I'd make an exception.'

George walked over to me and gave me a hearty slap on the back.

'No, seriously, Marc,' he said, 'well done. Next time invite the local papers, and get us some column inches.'

I watched the smile set into his face, as he turned away, took his bag and got into his Jaguar. He revved the engine a few times and wheel-spun out of the car park in a blaze of glory. It made my pathetic excuse for a vehicle look painfully inadequate. Useless piece of Italian junk. In all the excitement of the night before, I'd forgotten how spectacularly it had let me down. Perhaps

I should have listened to Ruth all along. But please don't tell anyone I said that.

Gloria went home and for a moment it was just me again, in this practice that had become more like home than my apartment these days. My flat was just a place to sleep, a pit stop to refuel in, a docking bay. I looked at the clock. It was almost half past six. Right on cue, Ruth burst through the door like a big ball of New Age energy.

'Hiya, Marc,' she said. 'Ready to go?'

My head turned. And froze.

'What have you done to your hair?'

Ruth laughed.

'Oh, I just thought I'd change things round a bit.'

'But it's *green*,' I said.

'Only a few strands of them,' she said, pointing to the streaks in her hair, 'two at the front, and one at the back.'

She flicked her head round so I could see it all.

'You'll never be taken seriously Ruth,' I said, '*we'll* never be taken seriously.'

'Speak for yourself,' she said snottily, 'you're a fine one to talk. Is that a Shiraz or a Cabernet?'

'Eh?'

'The splodges on your shirt,' she said. 'You know, Marc, you really should look into dry cleaning or we'll never be taken seriously.'

I walked over to the kitchen and put the kettle on.

'Can I have a tea?' she said. 'It's the white box with the pictures of dandelions on the front.'

'RUTH!' I said.

She stuck out her tongue.

'It's good for complexion,' she said, 'you should try it.'

As a punishment for looking so ridiculous I set Ruth finding quotes to get the car fixed. Preferably with a courtesy car.

The first patient was not what you would typically class as an emergency.

'What happened?' I said, as the owner reached into her cat carrier. She was a young American woman, newly married to a Brit and recently settled into the area.

'We were making soup,' she said, 'Heinz Cream of Tomato…'

'Right…' I said.

There was a soft sheepish meow, as out of the top of the carrier she lifted out a fluffy seven-month-old Ragdoll kitten.

'He was so pretty,' she said, 'I've ruined him.'

Rocky peered up at me.

Erin's face filled with red.

'I, er, take it that's not his natural colour?' I said.

'I told Davey not to leave the soup pan on the table. He licked the edge and tumbled in after.'

I tried to mask a smirk. It said 'Seal bi-colour' on the computer records. Rocky was bright neon orange.

'Does he come with a bread roll?'

In all emergencies it's important to keep your spirits up. In a stressful treatment room, a sense of humour helps to alleviate nerves and take a lid off the pressure. But there are some things you can't laugh about, and in some situations, it's hard to find some lightness, like Maggie for example, the next patient through the doors.

Maggie was an ancient Yorkie suffering from end-stage heart failure. Bob and Linda had been her caring and attentive owners for 17 years. She had the run of the house. They'd brush and groom her every day, and lay a rug down at the foot of their bed for her to sleep on. They were quiet, considerate people who'd been in and out of various different surgeries with Maggie for a long list of medical problems over the years. But in the last six months their visits had become increasingly frequent. They were resigned to the fact that Maggie was coming to the end of her life, and Gloria said that on each visit, she watched their shoulders sink a little bit lower than the last.

Yorkies come in two types of coats, a silky and a soft. Maggie was a beauty with a silky blue and tan coat, though the blue had lightened to a burnished steel as she'd aged, gracefully. Her muzzle was a pale grey and she had long lost much of her hearing and sight. She was slow and lethargic and there was a cloudy blue haze over her eyes. Her medication list was a similar length to my grandmother's.

Bob and Linda were in their sixties, and were sombre, quietly devout people of few words. When I picture them now, I see them in a garden, Linda kneeling by a rose bush, snipping off great big blooms in a floppy sun hat with a pair of secateurs, Bob somewhere in the background mowing wide stripes into the lawn. I want to call them 'slow', but they weren't 'slow' in intellect, just slow in judging others and slow to anger.

Bob and Linda knew that Maggie was coming to the end of her life and while they didn't want to prolong her suffering, they acted on an unswerving commitment to protect the sanctity of life.

When Maggie came in she was barely alive. She was coughing, her tummy was swollen and pear-shaped as fluid had accumulated around her liver in her abdomen. Her mouth was not a healthy pink and the vessels were congested with blood. I watched an irregular heartbeat in the jugular vein of her neck. Ruth and I rushed her straight through to the ward and put her in an oxygen tent. I carried her in my arms, limp and heavy, and laid her on the floor of the tent. The tent was to aid her breathing, and to help get more oxygen to the heart to ease the pain, but we urgently needed to take a further load off. Not a lot of people know this but the widely used explosive nitroglycerine can also be used in medicine to very effectively widen the blood vessels in the skin of the patient, having the effect of making the veins relax and widen. When blood vessels do this, they open up more space inside and create less resistance and congestion, which makes it easier for the heart to pump blood around the body. In humans the ointment is applied to the chest or thigh and absorbed through the skin into the bloodstream, in animals we apply it to the shaved areas of skin like the groin or armpit area.

Maggie's heartbeat was irregular as she lay, collapsed at the back of the tent. It was clear to both Ruth and I that we could perhaps prolong her life, but she would remain in considerable pain, and anything we could do would merely draw out her deterioration.

I left Ruth in the ward with Maggie, while I went to speak to Bob and Linda. They were hunched over in the waiting room, sat next to each other, almost in the same posture, elbows on knees, hands in hair. They looked up as I walked in. Bob was wearing a woollen jumper and had a mop of thinning blond hair. Linda had tight brown curly locks. I shuffled into the room, at a deliberate, sensitive pace. Linda raised her eyebrows at me, then lowered them slowly down when she saw the look on my face. There wasn't much I needed to say. I could see that they knew that. I took a chair from the opposite side of the room and placed it carefully down in the front of them. We sat there in silence for a while.

'I'm sorry,' I said, 'Maggie isn't going to pull through.'

I was expecting tears and quivering lips, but I think they both knew it was coming. Linda remained composed. I watched her pick up her hand and place it on her husband's knee. He placed his hand on top of hers.

'Did she… did she pass away?' she asked.

'No,' I said, 'not yet. I'm afraid Maggie is in considerable pain, and anything we try will just prolong her suffering. The best thing for her would be to let her go to sleep.'

I clasped my hands together.

'Absolutely not,' said Bob.

The words hung in the air.

He stared at the carpet. I didn't know quite what to say.

'Absolutely not,' he said again.

I leant forward in my chair.

Bob let go of Linda's hand and folded his arms.

'I understand how hard a decision like this can be –' I paused '– but Maggie is suffering.'

I looked at Linda's stoic gaze into nothingness.

'Mr Abraham, Linda and I are adamantly against euthanasia,' said Bob. 'Everything that lives is holy, all life is sacred.'

'I couldn't agree more,' I said, 'but Maggie is suffering from end-stage heart failure, she is in a great deal of pain.'

Bob looked at me with a righteous calm. 'We will not give our permission to end her life. We simply do not have that right.'

I sat back in my chair and took a moment.

'Do you want a few minutes to talk with your wife?' I said.

'No,' he said, 'that won't be necessary.'

'Maggie's condition will not improve, but at this rate she could suffer for days.'

'Mr Abraham, I think we have been clear enough.'

'Would you like to see Maggie?' I said.

'We do not give you our permission to end her life,' he said.

Linda clenched her hands.

Bob stood up from his chair.

'Mr Abraham, we would like to take our dog home.'

'She's in Intensive Care,' I said, 'we cannot let her go.'

'Where is she?' said Bob.

I looked him in the eyes and wondered whether to tell him or not. He might do something but he did have a right to know.

'Downstairs,' I said.

Bob didn't need to be invited. He walked clean out of the waiting room, down the corridor and disappeared down the stairs to the hospitalisation ward in the basement. Linda grabbed her handbag and headed after him with a mumbled 'Sorry.' It was less an apology, more a word to prepare for me for what was about to happen.

'Guys!' I called after them. 'Please do not interfere with Maggie's treatment.'

But it was too late for that. As I hurried down the corridor after them I could already hear the scuffle. Bob got to the oxygen tent and asked Ruth to step aside. He snatched Maggie from where she was lying and turned right around. She lay limply in his arms. What made this situation extremely dangerous was that some of the skin of the poor dog was smothered in the nitroglycerine ointment. The drug works by being absorbed through the dog's skin, which is why you need latex gloves to handle it. Bob took the dog without gloves and, in picking up the patient, his hands were now coated.

'Bob,' I said, 'Bob, now, put the dog back down.'

Nitroglycerine causes drowsiness and lethargy as it begins to work and affects the heart.

'Bob, listen to me, you need to put Maggie back down,' I said, 'I'm saying this for your own safety.'

Bob glowered at me.

I continued to try to talk him down, but I could see Bob wasn't listening. Ruth pulled out her telephone and announced she was going to call the police. That's when they made a dash for it. Linda pushed the bar on the fire exit doors that opened into the car park and the two of them ran to their car. Ruth dialled 999.

Bob and Linda were putting Maggie in the back of their Ford Escort. I ran up to the passenger's door and pleaded with Linda.

'The ointment Bill has on his hands could make him pass out at any second. Do not let him drive,' I said.

Linda stared straight ahead as Bob turned the ignition.

'Do *not* let him drive,' I pleaded with her. 'BOB!'

At that moment Ruth leapt on the bonnet. Ordinarily I wouldn't encourage her impulsive behaviour, but like the previous night with the shopping trolley and the hospital trip, she had a guile that saved our necks. In moments of drama, just like Clark Kent whipping off his spectacles, Ruth transforms into a fearless superhero. She stretched out her arms and legs like a starfish and just lay there on her stomach on the bonnet of their car, head to the side, like an eco-activist with a JCB. Her hands were splayed across the windscreen, palms blocking their view. Bob wound down the window.

'Get off my bonnet! You are causing criminal damage.'

I stood back and let Ruth do her thing.

'If you drive this vehicle you could do you and everyone else serious harm.'

'Get off my bonnet, this minute!'

Then, in the distance, we a heard first one siren, then

one more. The station had sent two cars. As Linda jumped out and tried to prise Ruth's hands from the windscreen, the panda cards arrived and blocked the exits, barricading in Bob, Linda and Maggie. Ruth got off their bonnet, the officers stepped out of their vehicles and one by one we all went back inside.

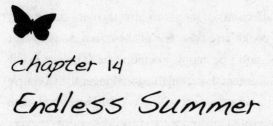

chapter 14

Endless Summer

I have this theory that there are two types of vets: the rooted – those who stay in the same veterinary practice for the majority of their careers, and if and when they move, it's only to join the other place down the road, and the journeymen – those who stay somewhere for a few years, and then one morning inevitably wake up with a feeling that it's time to move on. They pack their scrubs and their stethoscopes into a small handkerchief, tie it to the end of a pole and sling it over their shoulder in search of a new adventure. I'm of the latter group.

I've always envied those vets who manage to put their roots down. They build deep relationships with generations of fluffy and furry pet owners and look after their patients from cradle to grave. When you've worked in different practices, you quickly spot the rooted vets. They can't walk down a supermarket aisle without three different people talking to them. At Christmas they're the ones who get hundreds of cards, tins of shortcakes and biscuits and boxes of chocolates. When I see them in the waiting room, addressing each pet and owner by their first names with genuine affection, I stand on my own in the corner wishing I could have been one of them, but deep down I know I wouldn't be happy. I couldn't be. The fact is I've never been content doing anything for longer than a couple of years. It's been that way with every flat I've rented, with every housemate I've lived with, every car I've driven, every job I've had and every relationship I've been in. Some of us just grow up with shorter attention spans and bigger loftier dreams; it's just the way we're wired.

I kept my hands busy as a kid. My uncle used to call me 'prolific', a word I didn't really understand the meaning of, until someone explained it to me when I was older. When most children my age would choose to plonk themselves down in front of the television I would be copying out a picture of an animal from a book, or nipping out into the garden to look for animal tracks. My uncle was like a character from a Roald Dahl story, but not an evil one like Mr Twit, he was a kind sort, like the BFG. He was an exaggerated man, big, tall and happy, and he never lost his childhood sense of wonder. I heard a description the other day of people like that: they never forget that their adult world was built on top of the childish world under the stairs. That couldn't have been truer of my uncle. Whenever he found a quiet moment to slip away from my mum and dad, he'd come outside and stand beside me, encouraging me with a hand on my shoulder in whatever I was up to, and he'd make up elaborate stories about slugs and worms. He brought me all kinds of books about the natural world, and would take me to museums, but every so often he'd crouch down, put his big hand on my head, his fingers splayed out over my hair, look me in the eye and tell me in the wise old way that only the best grown-ups do, 'There is something you must always remember – we're human beings, not human doings.' My uncle was perceptive to spot that trait in me. I am no good at sitting still. I look enviously at the rooted, they're really good at 'being'. They're good at being married with kids and settling down, they're good at not tripping ahead of themselves, not chasing after the next big thing, that is only ever a step towards the next one. They're good at being content.

The only constant in my life has been restlessness, the urge to push on, to explore, and to find a new adventure. It was this urge that took me to Edinburgh, when my parents thought perhaps a university closer by would be better. And this same urge took me to Kentucky to work with the horses out there, to Herefordshire and a rural practice for a while, to the French Alps where I snowboarded, to Thailand where I dived, and eventually landed me here in Brighton.

I'd come back from hot and sunny Brazil where I had been working as a conservationist in the rainforests, and had moved in with a friend in Teddington, near Twickenham in London. I was working as a locum vet at a local practice. I'd swapped working with wildcats, ocelots and the spotless jaguarundis for trips to Tesco to pick up toilet roll and sit in front of episodes of *Cash in the Attic* on TV. Every day I'd wake up, brush my teeth, leave the front door and sit in traffic at the end of the road, wishing I could still hear the songs of the macaws and see jaguars asleep in the trees. Of all the chapters of my life, this one was one of the shortest. I love London, but it wasn't for me. It was like buying a jumper from a clothes shop without trying it on, wearing it out and thinking it looked good, but then getting home and realising it didn't. There were more clubs in London, more bars, and more young people per square metre than any other place I've ever been, but one night I couldn't sleep because I knew I'd had enough. It was two o'clock in the morning and I fumbled around on my bedside table for a pen. I still have the page in my notebook with my sleepyhead scrawl. I needed fresh air, crashing waves and strangers who actually talked to you. I wanted birdsong, hedgerows and walks in the woods. And when I woke up in the morning when my alarm clock went off, there was a single word written on my notebook: Brighton. And so that weekend I moved.

When I moved down to Brighton it was summer. It was probably the best summer of my life for three reasons – I like sunshine a lot; I am fond of beaches, even pebbly ones, and I like the sort of girls who love sunshine and pebbly beaches. I worked odd locum shifts and had time on my hands, time to kick off my shoes and slip on my flip-flops, time to meet people and enjoy life. It was sunny, there was always music playing, and a few months down the line, I was in love. I moved into a grand old neighbourhood. Like many British seaside towns, the Regency splendour had long gone, but a lively community had taken its place buzzing with flea markets, cafés and cool clothing stores and more than its fair share of eccentrics. It was a beautiful maze of pastel and white plaster buildings, each an apartment block, deli or seafront hotel, standing shoulder to shoulder like a line of wedding cakes. Walking to work, I would stop by the old sweet shop run by a curly-haired lady with a big red nose, it had shelves and shelves of pear drops and wine gums, Kola cubes and millions of jellied sweets, and I'd ask for a quarter of sherbet lemons and smile as she weighed them on the little scales and tip them into a paper bag. When I think back to my first summer all I can see is sunshine, all I can smell is Chanel No. 5 and all I can taste are those sherbert lemons. I've travelled around the world, I've surfed, partied and slept on some of the best beaches it has to offer, but with my hand on my heart I could say that there is nothing quite like Brighton in the summer. But that was my first summer in Brighton. And then one day I had that brilliant idea to set up an emergency veterinary surgery and work nights, six days a week, twelve months of the year, autumn, winter, spring and right the way through the most beautiful of the seasons – summer.

'Are you sick?' he said.

I was picking up a newspaper on the way back from work when I bumped into my old friend, Paul, in the street. He was munching on a sausage roll.

'Seriously, man, you look well pasty,' he said. 'Are you all right?'

I chose to deflect this question by asking after his girlfriend.

He looked at me with an idiotic stare. 'We broke up four months ago,' he said, 'where have you been?'

I made an apologetic face. 'I'm sorry,' I said, 'I've just been working a lot. Look, I'm sorry to hear about that.'

'Don't worry,' he said, 'I broke it off, seriously, dude, you look like a zombie.'

I looked down at my white arms, my white legs in my shorts, and to the white toes peeking out of my flip-flops.

'Ah! The good ol' British summer,' I said.

Before the words had even left my mouth, I knew it was a daft thing to say. Paul looked up at the heavens and back down at me with a puzzled look.

By British standards the sun was positively roasting, there wasn't a cloud in the sky. It had been that way for more than a couple of weeks, not that I had been awake at the times I could be appreciating it. Even with the curtains shut there'd be light pouring into my bedroom as I pulled the covers way up over my head and grumbled myself off to sleep. I looked round where he and I were standing. We were in a little patch of shade in the Lanes, a network of narrow streets and alleyways that is home to independent shops selling all types of things from vintage clothes to retro jewellery. The whole place smelt of summer, with wafts of sea air and ice creams and the coconut note of sun-tan lotions. It bubbled with the laughter of happy people in vests, shorts and skirts. Everyone was tanned. Everyone's hair seemed sunkissed. There was not a single person whose skin wasn't a shade of pink, red or brown. A freckly teenager with ginger hair cycled by on a BMX, even his skin was darker than mine.

'You don't get out much, these days, do you?' said Paul, looking at my arms.

And there and then it struck. In that encounter with Paul in the Lanes, my mind flicked back to my first summer in the city. And it was like someone had grabbed me by the sleeve and dragged me in front of a mirror. Because as I looked at my reflection I didn't recognise the person staring back. The earring was still there, as was the tattoo that peeked out of my T-shirt sleeve. But where had the fun, up-for-it, social Marc gone? All I could see was a pasty, veterinary hermit. Paul was looking me in the eyes.

'Really,' he said, in a semi-sympathetic way, though a bit like Jeremy Kyle, 'how you keeping?'

'Good,' I said, nodding my head a little too vigorously, 'yeah...good.'

It didn't sound all that convincing. There was Paul, tall, fit, tanned, smelling of a reasonably expensive aftershave and looking pretty content. He was probably on his way to a pub to meet a friend he'd already seen for a midweek pint. Maybe he was then off to meet a beautiful girl on the beach. And here was I.

'What's new?' he said.

My mind went suddenly blank. I couldn't think of anything to say. News...news...news...I couldn't remember the last time I'd met a fit girl on a beach. Or the last time I'd slapped on some aftershave before going anywhere other than work. I hadn't been away for a mini-break; I hadn't caught up with old friends. Nothing was new. My lifestyle wasn't really much to talk about. The only thing I did when I wasn't working was sleep, and I had bags under my eyes from not doing that particularly well. I wasn't in shape. I had developed a little belly. I ate the sort of food that asks you to remove packaging, pierce lid several times and leave to stand for a minute when done. I couldn't tell you what the inside of a gym looked like any more. My idea of a wild night was a can of Heineken in front of *Deal or No Deal*.

'The usual,' I said.

He nodded. It was the sort of nod that says *I thought as much*.

'Don't do that,' I said. 'Look, I'm sorry I've been off the radar a bit. I've got myself sucked into my work. When can we go for a beer?'

'What you doing tomorrow afternoon?' Paul asked.

I looked down at my wrist, as if there was something there. I didn't use a watch any more.

'What day is tomorrow again?' I asked.

'Sunday.'

I worked six days a week at the surgery. When I finished on Sunday morning at eight, we had a locum vet and locum nurse pair who would come in and take over. It gave Ruth and I the Sunday evening and following morning off, and then we were back at work at six o' clock on Monday night as usual. The hours being what they were, when I finished work on a Sunday I'd normally go straight to bed and sleep right the way to about six, at which point I'd meet a friend for a quiet beer in the pub, and climb into bed again just after midnight. I had to be more interesting. I had to stop being a hermit.

'Er, yes,' I said, 'in that case, I think I'm free.'

Paul smiled.

'Great. We're hitting it hard,' he said, 'it's my thirty-fourth birthday.'

I looked at him.

'Your birthday?' I said.

I couldn't believe I had forgotten.

'Since when did you celebrate a thirty-fourth?' I said. He snorted.

'It's a big deal, man, think about it. Thirty-four. I'll have lived longer than Jesus. My birthday's actually on Monday, so we're starting at twelve and drinking right the way through until midnight, seeing the big day in, then going for a swim in the sea.'

My mind went straight to sleep calculator. I could get two hours in in the morning, hang out for the night and if I slept right through Monday...

'Sounds great,' I said. 'Brilliant. Text me to tell me where you'll be.'

At work that evening all I could think about was how much I'd changed. It was good, I needed to change, everyone had told me that. As I put my scrubs on for duty I heard the voices of the partners from the previous place in my head, telling me I was too immature, that no one wanted to work with me, that I didn't know the first thing about business. I thought back to the frustrating phone call with my parents when Dad told me I needed to 'settle down'. They were right, but I wasn't ready to let the old Marc go, I still needed to let my hair down, what little of that there was. I realised that my 'big night out' was way too overdue when I couldn't stop thinking about it. I thought about everyone I knew grumbling about me behind my back. *Oh Marc, he's become so boring. What's up with Marc? Has anyone seen him?* And that just made me shudder. So I kept telling myself that I was going to turn up all high energy and show them how to have a good time. Show them that I hadn't lost it, I was still one of the funnest guys I know. I made a little pact with myself that I would be the last one there, whatever that took, even if it meant I was still swimming in the sea when the sun came up.

It was a fairly quiet night at the surgery, we had a few patients drop in, but none you would classify as actual emergencies, which was a good job, my mind was on other things. I must have bored everyone stupid. There was a boy called Anthony in my class at school who came to class one morning boasting that he'd got himself drunk on the weekend by drinking 16 cans of Shandy Bass that he'd bought from Superdrug. And as I talked about my 'big night out' with Ruth, I felt a bit like him. It wasn't cool. I didn't care. In fact, I was interested to see if she felt the same.

'Do you go out much?' I asked her.

Ruth laughed. 'Not since I've worked here,' she said.

We were sitting around in our makeshift lounge area. She picked at a strand of thread poking out of the sofa. It was pitch black outside. Another beautiful sunny day had been and gone, and we'd seen about 56 minutes of daylight between us.

'God,' I said, 'look at the pair of us.'

Suddenly something came over Ruth. She hopped up and threw me the remote control. 'Stick it on MTV Base and turn it up. Come on,' she said, raising her hands to the ceiling, 'it's the nightshift, and I'm in need of some fresh beats.'

I nearly fell off the sofa laughing.

Ruth cranked up the volume, as summery Euro-pop music blasted from the speakers, and shiny dancers leapt about a white screen. Ruth hopped about the floor, like she didn't have a care in the world, pulling off moves you'd never think were possible for a human being. I sat back on the sofa and smiled, eyes popping out of my head, and I discreetly edged the volume down when she wasn't looking to make sure we could still hear the telephone.

Paul's party started at a cosy little pub near the seafront. There wasn't a whiff of a chain pub or a gastro pub about it, you couldn't buy deep-fried Camembert or shiitake mushrooms or pumpkin risotto with shavings of aged Parmesan; it was scampi fries and pork scratchings or nothing. There was even a large wooden sign behind the bar with a hobgoblin swigging a tankard of ale carved into it – the caption below him read 'What's the matter, Lager-boy – afraid you might taste something?' The pub opened at twelve on the dot and Paul promised me they'd be queuing up outside from quarter to. I got back from the shift at nine and managed to squeeze a couple of hours of sleep in before having a quick shower and a shave, and digging out a clean white T-shirt. I arrived at the pub a little after the others on the grounds there was a chance some of our clients would be around, and I wasn't sure I wanted to be seen waiting in line for a pub to open. Paul had booked a couple of tables in the corner, within arm's reach of a computerised quiz machine, the establishment's single concession to the changing times.

'Mate,' said Paul jumping to his feet. 'Everybody, this is the famous Marc Abraham. Be gentle with him, he doesn't get out much.'

The table cheered. A frothy pint of beer was immediately thrust into my hands. The pub was full of faces I recognised and quite a few I didn't. And as the guys got up to greet me, I found myself beaming from ear-to-ear. It felt like a homecoming and I hadn't even realised I'd been away. I felt a little pride swelling in my chest as I talked about the practice Ruth and I had built out of nothing. I held my own when it came to swapping stories, serving up the tales of the dreadful practice car, the take-away menus and the gerbil woman, which had the table in stitches. We stayed at the pub for a couple of hours and reached that point where we either dig our heels in and set up camp or move on to somewhere else. And I was mightily relieved when Paul suggested we move outside so I could get some colour in my cheeks; one of the guys produced a Frisbee, and we trooped down to the beach, with a couple of carrier bags of trendy cider.

I closed my eyes and took in a big lungful of salty air. It was a totally stunning day, the sun was beating down and everyone was happy. Children ran round with ice cream dropping off their cones. Pensioners sat in stripy deckchairs and tutted at what some of the young people were wearing. Young people with their jeans slung low looked blankly at the pensioners and wondered why they were wearing jackets. The promenade was buzzing with huge queues for fish 'n' chips and even bigger ones for refreshments. Girls of all shapes and sizes sat around plastic picnic tables while their guys joined the monstrous queues at the bars and waited their turn to be served then came back with sloshing jugs of drink and stacks of plastic glasses. The beach was packed with the usual British holidaymakers and, Brighton being Brighton, also plenty of the city's alternative crowds. There were two large gay wedding parties taking photos up the steps, complete with cross-dressing vicars and page-dogs – two cute little English toy terriers in huge baby blue bows.

The beach at Brighton is big enough to accommo-date everyone, in different pockets of activity. Standing up by the road you could see it clearly enough to map it. The families had taken over the area nearest the pier. They

were the ones who'd arrived at the beach first and staked
their claim to the pebbles with their flags, windbreaks and
tents. The children were down by the water, screaming
and squealing as they ran in and out of the surf. The
further you walked away from the pier, the more diverse
the crowds became. First you met the couples, out for a
romantic afternoon, lying on towels, lying on each other,
doing what lovers do. Out from the couples were dark
outcrops of Goths, dressed from head to toe in black.
They were gathered around small smoky fires, like a scene
from *The Hobbit*, and lying stiff like boards listening to
their headphones. Near where we set up our camp a party
of students arrived with the components for a hi-fi stack.
They gaffer-taped a huge car battery to the top of the
stack and began to pump deafening reggae music from
an iPod; it travelled in waves across the beach. And like
moths to a flame it wasn't long before a party gathered
around them, smaller groups shuffling closer and closer
in, until an impromptu group of once-strangers were
singing Bob Marley at the top of their lungs, and barter-
ing sandwiches for cans of beer. Everyone brought their
own bottles and cans and the numbers swelled into an
outdoor beach party. And it wasn't long before we found
ourselves migrating over. To the strains of 'One Love' and
'I Shot the Sheriff' I slipped into my board-shorts,
grabbed a bottle of beer and charged into the sea.

chapter 15
Hanging in the Balance

The first thing they noticed when I got in to work was my face. It was hard to disguise. I couldn't exactly walk in wearing sunglasses and a balaclava and expect no one to be suspicious. It wasn't just my face, my whole head, neck, ears and nose were tender and pumping out heat like a radiator. My neck was sunburnt in a perfect 'V' where my T-shirt had stopped. My arms were the colour of Scottish salmon. From the moment the day staff saw me, they tipped back their heads and laughed their socks off, and they were still laughing when I walked straight past them and had reached the end of the corridor.

'Marc,' Gloria said trailing me to the common room, 'did you get stuck in the tanning machine?'

'It's not funny,' I said.

'It looks serious,' she said.

My head even hurt to shake.

'Is Ruth in yet?' I croaked.

'No,' said Gloria, 'not that I've seen.'

She paused and watched me a second. The mood changed. She was a little more sympathetic.

'What happened?' she said. 'Did you fall asleep?'

'Something like that,' I said.

Gloria walked over for a closer look. She pursed her lips and made an 'ooooh' sound.

'Ouch! Marc,' she said, 'do you want some cream? I've got some Sudocrem in my bag?'

'I'd take ibuprofen, if you've got some,' I said.

She screwed up her eyes and looked at me for an entire minute.

'What?' I said.

Gloria was reading my mind. 'Do I want to know what you've been up to?' she said.

I hung my head. 'I don't think you do,' I said, 'no.'

She tried to pull a disapproving face but cracked a little smile, turned around and pottered off to find something for my pain.

When Ruth arrived a few minutes later, she wasn't in a much better state. She had mentioned to me on Saturday that she and her boyfriend Rich might also be down at the beach, and so I'd told them if they saw us to come over to say hi, and somehow around six o'clock we all got swept up into the monster reggae party. There must have been 200 sun-worshippers dancing around the hi-fi, laughing and having fun, as you do so easily in summer. And as the night drew in we lay out on the beach and stared up the stars and danced in the moonlight. When we looked at our watches Paul's thirty-fourth birthday had arrived without us even knowing; there was a flurry of champagne and some people said their goodbyes and began to drift off home. But not Paul. Needless to say, I kept the promise I'd made to myself to be the last man standing. And the party did end with a dip in the sea, but that happened after the sun came up.

We were a mess. Ruth plonked her carrier bag down on the table. All sorts of alternative pills and herbs poured out on the table. It was like the contents of a witch doctor's medicine cupboard. There really was nothing to say, so she made a big mug of something and another for me. When we could talk, we did so with hushed voices to spare both the embarrassment of being overheard, and our heads.

'Ohhh!' I said, clutching my temple.

'Ughhh!' she replied.

'What time did you guys get back?' I asked.

She leant against the wooden table and gripped it with both hands. Her knuckles turned white for a second then went back to a pasty yellow. She arched her back, and dropped her head, like she was performing a dramatic yoga move. She sucked in a lungful of air and held it. When her head came back up again her eyes looked like they were swimming in the middle of her face. I reached across to the tub of Sudocrem that

Gloria had kindly brought in with the tablets, and a glass of water.

'Seven o'clock,' she said, finally exhaling and emptying her lungs, and she dipped her head back down again ready to suck in another deep breath. 'When we were leaving Rich insisted I made him bacon and egg when we got home. Poor sod had to go straight out to work.'

'What?' I said, dabbing a tender spot on my ears.

'Well, he should have done,' she said, 'in actual fact he passed out on the bus.'

I dipped my finger in the cream and drew a cooling line across my forehead. It was painful to the touch, and even though I was more than exhausted when I had finally made it to bed, and peeled off my clothes, I hadn't been able to get much sleep. I'd really only snatched a handful of hours since Saturday afternoon, and coupled with my toxic head, the evening's surgery was going to be a challenge. I'm not far off being atheist, but I sent up a mumbling, hungover prayer to God to have mercy on us. But I think he had an axe to grind.

'Call me if you need anything,' said Gloria, popping her head round the door.

'We will,' I said.

She stood there looking at Ruth and me, like a captain would look at two sea-sick sailors. 'You two! I'd keep this door shut if I was you. George is still around somewhere, and, you know, I think that's best. And open the window a crack. There's a strange brewery-type smell coming from somewhere.'

With that, Gloria shut the door behind her with a definite click. We heard her footsteps grow quieter as she walked down the corridor. I looked shamefully at Ruth and Ruth looked shamefully back. Was it really that obvious?

'Oh dear,' I said.

'Bollocks,' said Ruth under her breath, 'bollocks, bollocks, bollocks.'

I went off to brush my teeth again, and Ruth stamped her feet on the carpet in frustration.

Looking back on the shift, the problem was not that we had too much to do, it was the exact opposite. If we had been busy we would have kept on going. We would have had one of those all-out-war nights sponsored by Red Bull and adrenaline. We would have turned the music on, cranked open the windows and let in the balmy fresh air. Maybe we would have been so busy we would only have had enough time to snatch a passing look at pictures of the night before on Ruth's camera phone, before rushing off to see to another emergency. But sadly, none of that happened. At first there was a trickle of patients. Our first had heatstroke of all things. Jasper was a beautiful golden retriever. He was two and half years old, and had been left in the back of a Vauxhall Corsa. The owner said he'd left the passenger window open a crack, but it must have been the tiniest crack, and the car must have turned into an oven. Jasper's owner went to meet an old school friend for a light dinner out at the beach and, as is so easy to do when you're out having fun in the sunshine, he forgot how long they'd been there. When he got back to the car, Jasper was breathing frantically, making scary, noisy breaths. The moment his owner reached the car, Jasper vomited in the back all over the footwell. Prompt action almost certainly saved his life. I told them to drive immediately over with the air-conditioning cranked down low, and as soon as they got here we put him in a cool bath and took his temperature. Jasper's core temperature was a full seven degrees above the normal. The average for a healthy dog is 37–39 degrees Celsius. If his temperature had gone up by just one degree more he could have gone into a coma and his organs would have started shutting down. Thankfully, Jasper went on to make a full recovery, but the irony of a sunburned vet lecturing his owner on heatstroke was not lost on me. As soon as they'd left I went back to the Sudocrem pot and dabbed the cooling white cream over my ears and on the crown of my head, cursing my stupidity.

After Jasper, we had a little wait. Ruth and I sat out on the steps at the side of the building, watching the holidaymakers in the neighbourhood going from bar to bar.

There was that summer evening buzz in the air, but absolutely nothing inside me wanted to join in, all I could think about was the dull throb in my head. We talked about swings and roundabouts, how everything in life comes with a cost. Thinking about our situation, and the hours we worked, I talked about how there was nothing in me that wanted to go back to my student days when I had all the time in the world, but didn't know what to do with it, how I didn't envy the freedom I used to have, to do what I wanted when I wanted. I liked my life. I was enjoying the responsibility that comes with running a business. Sure, it cost me a bit of freedom, but it was just for a few years, and it came with its own rewards. We provided an invaluable service. And in the darker days you have to try to remember the faces of the people you'd helped. And then I realised it was time for another ibuprofen. We saw one or two more patients. A cat came in with a cut to her leg from the jagged edges of a tin can lid, she needed a stitch or two and a light bandage to prevent infection, and right after her was a four-year-old boxer with a grass seed lodged in his ear. After they left it was eleven o'clock, and the phone didn't ring for hours.

I woke sometime after three o'clock to pounding fists on the front door, yelling and shouting. I opened my eyelids but my eyes were blurry, and I couldn't make out a thing. I was sort of sitting upright but I was slouched in the chair, so my knees came out some way and my feet were flat on the floor. I felt about myself to find my bearings. The pounding moved to the window, and then I heard Ruth's sleepy voice.

'Marc!' she said. 'Marc!'

As I pulled my eyes into focus a number of things became immediately clear to me. First of all, the time. The digital screen of the DVD player said it was 3.15 am. The DVD menu screen was playing, and looping the same signature tune round and around and around. It was the *Star Wars* theme. I'd forgotten we had put a movie on, I must have slept right the way through it. The second thing I noticed was the mess across the carpet. By my left foot was an overturned bowl and in front of me were hundreds of crunched up Cool Original Doritos strewn across the carpet. And the last thing I noticed before I turned to the man at the window was the flashing red light on the answerphone. I screwed up my eyes and tried to read the number next to it. Was it a two or a four?

'Marc!' said Ruth, standing over me. 'Would you go?'

The number on the answerphone was nine.

'What the hell are you doing?' yelled the man at the door, a vein was popping out of his neck and his face was red. He shook his head. 'Were you having a sleepover?

A movie night? We've been calling and calling and calling for you for the last three hours.'

'I'm sorry,' I stuttered, still in a daze. 'Come in.'

I didn't know what else to say. The man was livid. He bounced up and down on the soles of his shoes on the welcome mat and clenched his hands, fishing for a more reasonable answer from me. But I didn't have one. There was no reasonable answer. We had simply fallen asleep. So the man and I ended up just staring at each other, eyeball-to-eyeball, exchanging blank looks until I blurted out, 'Ruth, will you prepare the consulting room?' and she shuffled back off down the corridor to get the table ready and to freshen up.

'I'm so sorry,' I said again and I looked about him for his pet, to try to gauge the severity of the situation. 'I really can only apologise. This has never happened before.'

The man glowered back at me. He was taking it all in, as if noting down all the details to write in a letter to the newspaper – my burnt red face, the dark bags under my eyes, my crumpled, creased scrubs that had doubled as my pyjamas. He shook his head and said, 'We'll talk about this later,' then he turned and walked quickly back to his car.

'This way,' he said.

I brushed the crumbs off my legs and hurried after him.

In the back of Mr Morris's Ford Mondeo lay Stock, a beautiful Bernese mountain dog, wrapped in a thick blue blanket.

'He collapsed,' said Mr Morris. 'He became suddenly very dizzy, stumbled and then fell over. My wife and I were lying in bed when we were woken by the sound of Stocky stumbling around the bedroom. He let out a painful yelp and hit the deck.'

Mr Morris told me how his wife had jumped out of bed and turned on the lights to investigate and that was when they noticed Stock couldn't get up. He was paralysed in the front two legs. That was just after midnight. His eyes went wide again.

'We've been ringing you since then. What time is it now?' he said.

'Three fifteen,' I replied.

'That was over three hours ago,' he said.

I swallowed. 'Please, try to remain calm,' I said.

'It's hard to remain calm when I couldn't get hold of you!' he yelled. 'This could be a matter of life and death. We looked online, we did our research. Some dogs died because they hadn't been treated soon enough.'

Mr Morris pointed to a metal bowl in the back of the car, then to the blanket they'd put around him to keep him warm, as if to make a point. They'd done all they could, any responsibility for the dog's condition was being placed squarely at my feet. Mr Morris kept turning around on the spot. He was understandably worked up and when he talked it came out in bursts like machine-gun fire, and the barrel was pointed at me.

'There's fresh water there, look…I had to bang on your windows…why didn't you hear the phone?'

I put a hand on his shoulder. 'I know, Mr Morris, I'm sorry,' I said. 'Come on, let's try to help your dog as quickly and calmly as we can, and we can talk about the rest of it later…'

While they waited by the phone, Mr Morris's wife had been searching on the Internet for help, visiting Wikipedia and all sorts of forums for pet owners and pet experts. While she was at the computer, Mr Morris crouched down by the dog, and just kept talking and reassuring. *It's okay, Stock, you're going to be all right.* There's lots of information available on the Internet and some of it is helpful but more often than not information can be misleading or totally incorrect, owners will naturally work themselves up by misdiagnosing all sorts of problems, and they come to their vet in a hot panic when often the situation presenting is far more routine. In this case, however, the advice that they had found – the blanket and the water – was helpful; collapse is a very serious condition and it is absolutely paramount that the dog is seen to as quickly as possible, and treated within 24 hours. Collapse is defined medically as a sudden loss of strength that causes a dog to fall, and from which he is unable to get back up again. It's akin to a stroke in a human, but it's complicated to diagnose the underlying cause of the symptoms. It's either triggered by a major disorder of the nervous, muscular skeleton, circulation or respiratory system, and pinpointing it can require many tests in a process of elimination. I could see from Stock's glassy eyes and look of confusion on his face that while he was still conscious, he was barely hanging on. He wasn't responding to sound or touch, but was shaking uncontrollably.

I asked Mr Morris to help me lift him and I carried him inside. Bernese are big heavy dogs, they were originally farm dogs that would drive dairy cattle huge distances, so are built for strength and agility. I took Stock in my arms, carried him across the tarmac and brought him straight into the consulting room. When we laid him down on the table, I unwrapped him from his blankety cocoon. And as he lay there, shivering in his beautiful tricolour coat, it became clear to me that the disorder hadn't just affected Stock's legs, like Mr Morris had told me, he was paralysed from the neck down. The situation was incredibly serious. I pulled up a plastic chair and motioned Mr Morris to sit down. As he sat I squatted down next to him, so we were looking eye-to-eye.

'Mr Morris,' I said, 'we need to take Stock into intensive care.'

At first Mr Morris was totally expressionless, then he scowled a little, looked at the floor and I watched his eyes fill up with tears. He wiped them away with a finger.

'He's presenting with what looks like paralysis,' I told him, 'but he doesn't appear to be in much pain. We need to conduct some tests to find out what has triggered it before we can do anything else.'

Mr Morris clenched his fist into a ball, and then unclenched it again. When he looked up, the surface of his eyes were glazed.

'What is it?' he said, swallowing. 'Tell me what's wrong.'

'He's in the best hands now,' I said. 'I'm afraid it's a process of elimination. We'll conduct some tests immediately and make sure he's comfortable. The best thing is if we can keep in touch by telephone. Give Ruth your number, and you've got ours. Please believe me when I say we're going to give him the best possible care.'

It was devastating to see him in his mixture of fear and frustration, and he had someone to pin the frustration on – me. You could see how little he trusted us when he left the practice and got back into his car. There was nothing we could do to change that, but do our jobs. I had never fallen asleep on duty before, and it called my whole decision to start the surgery into question, though now wasn't the time to think about that. I stood at the window, with my hands in my pockets, and

I watched him reverse out of his parking space, turn the corner out and disappear up the road. When I turned around, Ruth was sitting down, with her face in her hands. Big, wet tears broke out of the corners of her eyes and rolled down her cheeks. A lump grew up in the back of my throat. I wandered over to Ruth.

'Come on,' I said, 'there's only one thing for it.'

I held out my hand and pulled her up.

We turned to the table where Stock was lying and Ruth put on her gloves.

And deep down I despised myself.

George summoned me to the practice an hour and a half earlier than I would normally have arrived. Usually his text messages were light and jovial, ending with a 'love George' or a 'G x' this one just said – MARC. CAN YOU COME IN AND SEE ME AT 4.30? No sign off. No kiss. No silly little joke at the end. I immediately felt sick. I had some explaining to do. In the six months I had been there I had only seen a few glimpses of the partners. Because of the different hours we kept, we had few interactions. Every other month we had a two-hour meeting to discuss housekeeping matters and as a forum to swap ideas, and share our gripes about the handovers, cleanliness and the short supply of toilet rolls. When I thought about it, the only sides of George I had seen were the diligent well-loved veterinarian and the jovial entertainer. I'd never seen him angry, upset or disappointed, so I wasn't quite sure what to expect when I arrived. But my mind thrashed about, splashing in the puddles of a sea of different scenarios. What if they told me there and then that it was over? That that was it? What if I had blown it? In a weird way our previous night's unprofessionalism was wholly tangled up with the fate of the Bernese mountain dog. The biggest thing was that the whole affair made me ask much more existential questions. Everywhere I looked I couldn't get Stock's face out of my mind. An image of him lying on the consulting room table, shaking with fear. Was I up to it? Could I handle the responsibility? Maybe the partners at the old practice were right. Perhaps I was too immature.

The early tests we'd performed on Stock had suggested that a fibrocartilaginous embolism was likely, an infarction of the spinal column. It's caused by a shifting piece of cartilage. It's an incredibly serious condition: when the blood supply is cut, a section of the spinal cord dies, and the dog becomes paralysed in one or more limbs. The damage is permanent, so any treatment we perform is limited in its effects. I couldn't help but think that if we'd got to Stock earlier we may have had a chance to contain the paralysis. He'd lost mobility in both of his back legs.

George wasn't the only one who had texted me. There was a short one from Paul. It said – GREAT

NIGHT. WELCOME BACK. And there was one from Mum that I couldn't bear to open. I turned my phone over so it was facedown on the dresser. And lay in bed, so frustrated with myself. I spent a little longer in the bathroom than normal, staring in the mirror. If they asked me to resign, I would without a question. At least my face wasn't throbbing any more, though it was still lobster pink. What was I going to tell Dad if they shut us down? Would I make up some excuse about the practice having some funding pulled, or the partners going in with another surgery and making ours redundant? Or should I just tell him the truth? I threw it all away for a party on the beach that I now couldn't even really remember. I played the conversation out in my head as I squirted a dollop of shaving foam into my palm and worked it in little circles about my face.

'Dad,' I said to the pink man in the mirror, 'it's me.'

I picked up my razor and sloshed it around in the water.

'You were right all along,' I said, 'I need to settle down.'

I shaved more meticulously than normal, and made sure the basin was spotless as the water whirlpooled and disappeared down the plughole with a burp. I unhooked a clean button-up shirt from the wardrobe, and sat on the end of my bed as I laced up a pair of smart black shoes, so shiny I could see my face in them. *All right*, I said to myself, *I've made my bed*.

I was ready to be fired.

'Would you like a cup of tea?' asked George.

'No, thanks,' I replied.

I noticed my hands were shaking. I clasped them together under the table. We were sitting in his office, which was a little room at the end of the corridor with a huge window. He had photographs of his family all over his desk. Framed certificates on the walls. A stack of car magazines. This was the office of a well-respected, responsible man.

'I imagine you know why I called you in early. I had a phone call today from a Mr Morris,' he said.

I looked down at the table.

'How's the dog?' I said. 'We carried out tests.'

'We're keeping him in intensive care. He has a fibro-cartilaginous embolism, as you suspected.'

I nodded. 'Before you say anything,' I said, 'I want you to know that I totally accept your decision and if you decide that—'

George raised his hand and cut me off.

'Marc. Edward and I had a chat about it this afternoon,' he said. 'Now I know you probably think that if you'd gotten to him sooner you could have prevented it spreading. Well, you couldn't have done anything more than you did. I told Mr Morris that too.'

I folded and unfolded my hands under the table.

'What I was about to say earlier—' I said, then cut myself off. 'Is it both back legs?'

'Both back legs,' he confirmed. 'They've been in to see him this afternoon, and both Mr Morris and his wife were understandably upset.'

'George, I want to apologise,' I said. 'If you want to let me go I—'

'Don't apologise to me, Marc,' he said. 'I think you know how serious it was. And I'm sure you know what you need to do. I think you've done an amazing job so far. We've all had moments when we've dropped the ball. It was perhaps unfortunate that both and you and Ruth chose the same moment to drop them. I told Mr Morris that we wouldn't be charging him for the time he's spent with us. So I think we've been spared the letter to the newspaper.'

'What?' I said, rocking back in my chair. 'Are you sure you don't want to fire me?'

George laughed. 'Of course not,' he said. 'Why would I ever do that? You fell asleep. We've all fallen asleep before. I could never work the hours you do.'

'Oh, thank you,' I said. 'That's such a relief. I'm so sorry.'

George got up from his chair and stuck out his hand. 'Go thou and sin no more,' he said, looking around my face. 'Now, do you want some cream for that nasty burn of yours?'

And he broke into a toothy grin.

For the whole of the next week, I felt like I'd been let out of jail. It was a time to reflect on where I was going and what I was doing. I had been given another chance, and I wasn't going to blow it. After Stock was released from intensive care, every morning after surgery finished I climbed into the Cinquecento and drove over to the Morrises' house. They lived in a cute little cottage on the outskirts of Brighton, with a huge, long garden that stretched all the way down to rolling fields. Stock used to be such an active dog, they'd go on walks along the hedgerows to a favourite little copse of trees, and Stock would chase rabbits and squirrels and wear himself out in the fresh air. Stock had stayed at the surgery for four days, and when he was finally brought home he needed constant nursing care and supervision. The Morrises were both retired so they had all the time it needed to lovingly care for him. Every few hours they rolled him onto his tummy and did physical therapy on his back legs, moving them backwards and forwards to encourage mobility. For everyone involved it was emotionally very tough. The living room had a huge glass window that looked out onto the garden, down to the fields, hedgerows and the favourite little copse. Stock lay there with his chin on the carpet making longing eyes at the world outside he couldn't reach. He had very little movement on his right side too. He was a prisoner in his own body, attempting to wag his tail like a white flag every time they came over. He was heavy to lift, but the Morrises moved him every so often so he could see different parts of the house. He used to love lying in the sunlight, and he barked when they carried him into direct beams of light, where it was cosy and warm. It wasn't just lifting and physical therapy, Stock needed constant supervision, and the Morrises took it in turns to help. There were several loads of laundry do to each day, washing his blankets, sheets and rugs. And at night Mr Morris set his alarm clock for three-hourly intervals, and he'd get out of bed and put on his slippers to go down to Stock, roll him onto his belly and move his hind legs backwards and forwards just as the therapist told them.

It can be so discouraging when you care so much and do so much therapy but see little physical improvement, and it's particularly hard when everything you do seems incapable of bringing any joy. I dropped by every day and spent an hour with them, asking them how they were holding up and talking through the different therapy options. As a vet you sometimes have an almost spiritual role to play. Whether you asked to be or not, you're a spokesman for the animal kingdom, so in a weird way, my being there to encourage them showed Stock's appreciation, on his behalf. I tried to keep their hope alive, by telling them how many dogs I'd seen that had regained some level of motor function and had gone on to lead an otherwise normal life. Over the weeks they tried all sorts of things; acupuncture didn't seem to have much effect, but hydrotherapy really seemed to work. Stock put his heart and soul into it, kicking his legs as the trainer supported him underneath. They took him swimming every week; every week he went for it and each week he grew stronger. And one weekend when they came home, they lay him down on the grass. Mrs Morris walked back towards the house and squatted down about thirty feet away. At first, Stock just lay there. Then after a minute or two, he brought his legs in and stood up. Stock staggered about four or five steps then lay down, paused for a minute then tried again, bringing his legs in and standing on his own. He wobbled another five steps towards her, he was veering to one side, but he was actually walking again. Mrs Morris burst into tears.

A month or two later an email popped into my inbox. It had been sent by Mr Morris when they had returned from the neurologist, who couldn't get over Stock's progress. Apparently the neurologist had called in his colleagues to make sure he wasn't hallucinating. Now Stock even retrieves things they throw for him. I clicked on the email's attachment and opened up a full screen shot of Stock lying on his belly in the garden. His tongue was hanging and there was a squeaky bone in the short grass in front of him. And in a funny green font, with a fake paw print next to it, it said, 'Thank you.'

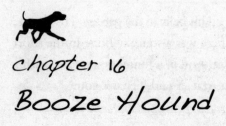

chapter 16
Booze Hound

When I was 15 our class was sent on a week of 'work experience'. I write this phrase in inverted commas, because I always failed to see how a week sitting around, twiddling thumbs, photocopying things that probably didn't need to be photocopied or reordering bookshelves in order of publication can ever be classed as experience of actual 'work'. It seems to me that in any profession there are a list of jobs that are not performed by anyone other than people on work experience, to the extent that the firm of accountants that I was assigned to had a work experience folder in their filing cabinet with lists of unseemly jobs for whoever was given the dubious honour of filling that role for the week. We all returned to our school-desks the following week and filled the class in on what we had been up to. Work experience is probably the single biggest reason why at the end of college or university so many students are desperate to flee to countries around the world, drink beer and refuse to wash their clothes under the proviso that this is a 'gap year'. I did however share a table with Thomas White, who spent his work experience at a marine biology institute, in a submarine. He was a nerdy computer kid, and I had never had cause to be jealous of him before, but when he got out his photographs, I cursed the fact that my dad was friends with Steele, Land & Partners and not Steve Zissou.

I was determined to give Dan some stories to share with his classmates. Dan was Fern's nephew. He had come in a few weeks before to discuss doing work experience with us and seemed keen enough, so I was happy to take him on. However, he was what you might call a proper partier, and true to form arrived hungover. He was drinking from a can of Coca-Cola.

'Me and my friends call it a red ambulance,' he said.

'What's that?' I said.

'Red Ambulance, the best hangover cure,' he said.

'You've studied biology and chemistry and that's the best hangover cure you can come up with?' I said.

Dan grinned. 'There's fourteen teaspoons of sugar in each can,' he said. 'That should do the trick. Why, what do you use?'

'Heineken,' I said.

He laughed.

Then I looked at him.

'Hang on, how can you still be hungover at 6 pm?' I said.

Dan smirked.

'I only just got up.'

*

Dan was one of those 17-year-olds who thinks he knows everything, on the grounds that he now shaved at least once a week (though not very well, it had to be said) and so had graduated into adulthood. He turned up at the practice in a navy blue hoodie with his nickname 'Danza' written across the back, and his hair immaculately spiked like a hedgehog.

'Change into scrubs,' I said, 'Ruth will show you where to find them.'

Dan played prop in rugby, and his shoulders almost touched both walls of the corridor as he went to the cloakroom to pick up his outfit. He was wearing a pair of hi-tops – those trainers that basketball players and hip-hop acts from the 1980s wear that come up to your ankle. 'You're not in a boy band, Dan,' I told him, in a tone that sounded like my mother. He walked back into the consulting room decked out in surgical scrubs, grinning like he'd just been given the ultimate fancy dress costume. I was just waiting for him to ask me if he could keep it when he was done. I rolled my eyes, knowing full well I would have done the same at his age. And when he held up his palm and said, 'High five,' I intentionally left him hanging.

Ruth came into the consulting room, with a list of patients on her clipboard.

'You've got a cocker spaniel called Max,' she said.

'Sweet,' I said, 'bring him in.'

Why did I say 'sweet'? I never usually said words like 'sweet' or 'dude' but I guess that's what hanging out with teenagers does to you.

Max staggered into the treatment room. He was a two-year-old cocker spaniel with a beautiful liver and tan coat, but he could barely stand up on his own four feet. Max's owner was a mumsy woman in her fifties. She was the outdoors type with trendy wellies, a quilted gilet and a string of pearls around her neck. Hers was the Range Rover parked up outside that we'd watch pull into the car park and take a few goes to reverse into a space. I held out my hand.

'Marc,' I said, introducing myself.

'Joan,' she replied.

'I hope you don't mind if Dan watches. He's on work experience.'

Joan nodded. We got to work.

Max was incredibly bloated. He looked like he'd been inflated with a bicycle pump. Even his cheeks were bloated. He staggered over to the wall and flopped down.

'Uh-oh,' I said.

'Is he pissed?' Dan piped up. 'He looks pissed.'

I threw Dan a glare, he covered his big mouth with his hand, in an 'oops' kind of way.

'I'm sorry,' I said to Joan, 'he's not been here very long.'

I turned back to her dog. 'He's very bloated, isn't he? What's the matter with Max?'

'Have a smell,' she said.

I knelt down beside her dog and even when I was halfway down I could smell the fumes rising up. There is no other way of putting it, Max reeked of booze.

'Whoa,' I said. 'What did he do?'

'He's drunk like a sailor on his first leave,' she said.

Dan made an I-told-you-so-face.

'He'll eat anything,' Joan said. 'I was baking a batch of little rolls and left them up on the table. That was at four thirty. Then I went out to pick up our youngest from violin. When I got back, Max had eaten half a kilo of fresh yeast dough.'

'Which fermented in his stomach,' I said.

If you've ever baked bread, you'll know that the dough likes a warm, moist place to rise. A dog's stomach is a nice warm, moist place and the dough can expand to several times its original size, which stretches the stomach and causes pain. It rises as the yeast ferments. The fermentation results in alcohol, which causes toxicity. Not only is this uncomfortable, it can be incredibly dangerous too.

'I Googled it,' said Joan, 'and came straight here.'

At that moment Max burped. It was a loud, almost human belch. The burps were what you'd expect from a drunk tramp on a bench.

'He's been doing that on the drive over,' said Joan. Then, dropping her voice to a whisper, added, 'And farts.'

'Wow,' said Dan, 'that's impressive.'

'The farts smell of baked bread,' she said, 'like you're at an actual bakery.'

I tried to remain professional, but I couldn't help but smile.

'Is it serious?' asked Joan.

'He'll be in a lot of discomfort. And, when it comes to ingestion toxicity it can be dangerous,' I said, 'but from what you're saying, with the amount of dough he has eaten, he's going to be okay. We can either give him something to induce vomiting or wait for the bread to work its way out.'

Joan nodded.

'We should give him something for his symptoms though. His stomach's going to be hurting. Do you have any Pepto Bismol?' I said.

Dan's face lit up with a big broad grin.

'Pink ambulance,' he said.

'What?' said Joan.

'Er,' he said, a little sheepishly, 'my friends call it the pink ambulance.'

Joan nodded along, though she had no idea what he was talking about. I was beginning to seriously wonder whether saying yes to Fern was the brightest thing to do.

*

The surgery was quiet, which was something of a relief. It was enough of a job just making sure Dan wasn't getting up to mischief, but it meant that we had a lot of time to sit and chat. Dan was a real talker, which though wearing, was a relief, as to my mind there's nothing worse than constantly having to think of how to keep a conversation going. Ruth, Dan and I sat around in the rest area and talked everything there was to talk about, with a little MTV in the background. We'd talked TV shows and sitcoms, Ruth had a book of yoga poses and she and Dan tried the scorpion and the reverse warrior, while R 'n' B hour blared in the background. Ruth asked Dan leading questions about his aunt, like 'So, is she single?' and 'Do you know if she has her eye on anyone?' whilst I tried to steer conversation elsewhere by asking him questions on every subject from *Baywatch* to Banksy, and somewhere along the line I mentioned studying at Edinburgh. Dan was slouching on the sofa, hi-tops on the table, munching from a bag of Doritos.

'What was it like?' asked Dan.

'Was what like?' I said.

He pushed the bag of crisps in my direction.

'Vet school?' he said. 'Did you always know you wanted to do this?'

'Be a vet?' I said. 'Yes, but I wanted to work with big animals, at first.'

'Like what?' he said.

'Well, I spent sometime in Kentucky, with race horses. That was interesting. But, I don't know, I was never great with farm animals at vet school.'

'What do you mean?' he said.

Ruth was doing a wheel pose. This is when you bend your back over so your tummy is in the air, your hands are flat on the floor, and your head is upside down.

'Tell him about the cow,' said a strained voice from her red face.

I rolled my eyes. Dan smiled.

'What happened with the cow?' he said.

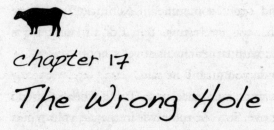

chapter 17
The Wrong Hole

There is a confession I feel I must make: in my youth I was a little like Dan. I applied myself to studying but I also appreciated that going to university was as much about living away from home for the first time, and everything that entails. When I first arrived at university, I was a little green behind the ears. The experiences of my first night should give you some indication of what I mean.

My arrival was fairly typical. I remained composed as I waved goodbye to my parents and unpacked what few boxes I had. There was flyer tucked under my door inviting me to a welcome night in the bar in my halls of residence. I decided to be fashionably late, so I wasn't the loner at the bar, and when I got there the evening was in full swing. There were hundreds of nervous new people asking the same questions time and time again like 'What are you studying?' and 'Where do you come from?', all huddled around like sheep and being super nice and polite. This was, believe it or not, my first proper experience of adult drinking. I strode straight up to the bar in the way Clint Eastwood might enter a saloon and ordered myself a Malibu and pineapple because I'd seen my sister do that, and when she did it she sounded quite cool. As I returned to my table full of rugby playing Scottish freshers, I learnt pretty quickly that there were more masculine drinks available for an English geeky first-time drinker. I soon found my feet and even found myself chatting to some girls at the bar. Things were looking up.

It was in the middle term of my first year that we were each sent out on placements to work with veterinary practices in Midlothian. I was down to work in a rural village practice, which primarily worked with farm animals. I had only lived in London and Edinburgh at that point, so my experience with the countryside had been limited to family holidays in Devon and Somerset, where the closest I had been to a cow or a sheep was as close as any typical rambler gets.

I was dropped at the practice where I would spend the week, bright-eyed and excited. Not knowing quite what to expect, I had made myself a packed lunch of cheese and pickle sandwiches, but in the taxi ride over I realised that I had somewhat overlooked breakfast so I took a punt that there would at least be a newsagent nearby that I could visit for a packet of Quavers, and wolfed them down. The taxi, however, drove through countless windy lanes, that all looked exactly like the last, and pulled up at this meagre-looking cottage with an oversized sign, with not so much as a pub or post office for miles. I was met by an elderly vet at the door with bushes of grey hair covering 50 per cent of his face. His name was Terry. Terry wasn't in scrubs and white tennis shoes, which are nowadays my working wardrobe, he was dressed in a tweedy jacket with a soft-checked shirt topped off with a flat cap. He looked like he kept whippets. I looked down at my shiny blue scrubs and wondered why I hadn't been warned about the dress code. The vet looked at his watch as if to make a point. It was barely nine o'clock.

'We country bumpkins keep different time to you soft city folk,' he said. 'Get in for eight in future. You ready to go?'

Soft city folk? I nodded keenly.

'Pleased to meet you, sir,' I said.

He grumbled something in reply.

I clambered into his Land Rover that was splattered with mud right up to the roof. The front windscreen looked like it had been covered by a few mugfuls of Bovril, with a semi-circle of visibility that the windscreen wipers had cleared. I made small talk and asked about the size of the village, the size of his caseload, and if there were any good pubs in the area. Terry didn't say very much to me. He grunted his replies, and I started to develop a theory that he didn't have much time for the

English, especially those from London. And when he did ask me questions I found myself shifting uncomfortably.

'Have they taught you much about cows?' he asked.

'Cows?' I said.

'Cows. You know, they go moo.'

I couldn't tell if he was joking with me, so I just made a sort of snorty laugh.

'I suppose I know a fair amount,' I said.

'All right, here we are,' he said, 'let's find out, then.'

We pulled up at a dairy farm. There were hundreds if not thousands of Friesian cows, dotted around the surrounding hills. It looked like a still from a Müller yoghurt commercial. The ground was muddy with trac-tor tread and littered with deep ruts now filled with dirty brown, sometimes oily puddles. Terry swung open the Land Rover door and squelched onto the ground. I shook my head as I tried to find somewhere soft to land but slurped into the mud up to my ankles.

'I see you've brought George Clooney,' said the dairy farmer when we walked into the shed. I hoped it was a reference to my good looks but it was probably a refer-ence to my immaculate blue scrubs, which was more suited to *ER* than a filthy cattle shed. The farmer sat on a barrel and looked me up and down.

Terry rolled his eyes. 'He's with us for a week. Go on, Marc, you do this one,' he said.

I had expected that I'd be getting my hands dirty at some point during the week, but not in the first half-hour. I stepped forward. Terry and the farmer raised their eyebrows.

'Pleased to meet you,' I said. 'What are we here for then?'

The farmer looked at me and said, 'I want to know if she's pregnant.'

'Pregnant?' I said, gritting my teeth. 'Cool. Well, let's see.'

I looked at Terry for some sort of cue, but he just stared right back at me.

'I need to get a few things from the car,' I said.

Terry threw me the keys and took a seat on a hay bale next to the farmer. I trudged out of the shed. I didn't turn back to see their faces but I'm sure he shook his head as I walked away.

I wasn't quite sure what I needed from the car, this was a cunning stalling tactic. The trek back bought me some crucial minutes to think things through. I had been at the husbandry lectures, and I knew we had been taught about this, I just had to find the appropriate place in my memory where I had stored the information. We had been through everything theoretically in the class-room and I knew my way round a cow, at least, a nice black-and-white diagram of a cow, but learning some-thing on paper in a light, state-of-the-art lecture facility in Edinburgh, is very different from actually doing it in practise on a squelchy farm in the countryside, especially when it's a procedure like this. Pregnancy. Cow pregnancy. I ran through the lectures in my head, mentally going over the notes, visualising the diagrams. There it was. To diagnose bovine pregnancy or check for an infection, you've got to reach into a cow's rectum and feel for the uterus, ovaries and Fallopian tubes. There's no substitute for getting up to your elbows in warm, gooey innards. *This is just a test to see what I'm made of*, I thought to myself, *but one thing I'm not is squeamish*. When I got to the Land Rover I looked inside the medicine bag for arm-length rubber gloves. Then I closed my eyes and muttered a prayer.

I took a deep breath before I stepped back into the cow shed. My heart was literally pounding; I'm sure the farmer's wife could hear it from the kitchen. I stood outside, just out of sight. Terry and the farmer were chuckling. When I stepped in, they fell silent.

'Okay,' I said, rolling the left sleeve of my shirt above the elbow, 'you all right?'

The two of them nodded.

'Get on with it,' said Terry.

The cow was huge. I approached it slowly from behind. Her stomach was massive. Her tail swished from side to side. I shuffled slowly forward so as not to startle or frighten her and very gently placed my right hand on her back. Her tail swished from side to side again. Was that a happy swish, an angry swish or a mildly irritated swish? My mind started to race. How would I know what to feel for? I mean, what do ovaries, cow ovaries, feel like? How on earth do they expect you to learn this kind of thing in a lecture hall anyway? I rested my head on my right arm as I felt around with my left, my gloved hand patting down directly below the tail. I went further and further down until I found the hole and inserted my hand. I went in as far as my elbow, the warm gooey innards pressing against my skin. I felt a surge of adrenaline, my heart was pumping. I had my arm in her rectum. And then I felt a hand on my shoulder. I looked round to see the farmer with his head in his hands. To see Terry's hand on my shoulder. I followed it up his tweed jacket to his face. Terry shook his head.

'That's the wrong hole, my boy,' he said.

He looked so disappointed with me. And I stepped back, and he stepped up, and the farmer patted the vacant hay bale next to him, and that more or less marked the beginning and the end of my time as a large animal vet.

Dan and Ruth were doubled up on the floor laughing.

'Oh, you can laugh, Dan,' I said, 'but don't think you're gonna get off lightly.'

I reached across to give him a playful slap.

'Don't come anywhere near me with those hands,' he said, grabbing my wrist, 'we don't know where they've been.'

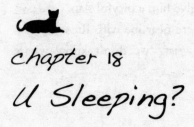

chapter 18
U Sleeping?

I was lying in bed when my phone beeped. For some reason I had it on one of those pointless alien ring tones that all mobile phones seem to have these days, which is never something you really want to wake up to.

> From: Mum - Wed 11:45 am
> R U SLEEPING?

I read it, stared at it, read it again. It was only three words but when you're in a sleepy stupor, it takes a moment to get your bearings. R U SLEEPING? It wasn't that I didn't understand the message I just couldn't comprehend what would possess anyone to send it. Come on, Mum, what do you think? I rolled over and dragged a swathe of duvet over my head. Twenty minutes later the second one arrived.

> From: Mum - Wed 12:03 pm
> R U SLEEPING? RSVP

U SLEEPING?

I picked up my phone and texted back. I WAS!! EVERY-THING OKAY?

> From: Mum - Wed 12:07 pm
> NO NEED TO BE SHORT. NOTHING URGENT.

I went back to sleep.

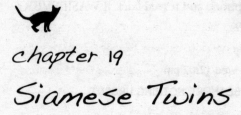

chapter 19

Siamese Twins

'No, Fern, I can assure you, Dan has been very helpful,' I said.

'Oh good,' she said, 'I wasn't sure.'

I shooed Ruth away with my hand. She kept listening in and grinning. I made a gesture with my hand and encouraged her out of the office.

'Sorry, Fern, I didn't catch that,' I said, swinging back on my chair. I had Blu-tacked a picture of the Arsenal football team to the wall to brighten up the space above my desk. I didn't have much tack so the picture kept falling off. I put a good amount of pressure on each of the corners with my thumb.

'Do you think he'd make a good vet?' she asked.

'He reminds me a lot of how I was at his age.'

'I should tell that to his mother,' Fern said, 'he hasn't always had what you would call a glittering school record.'

'Neither did I,' I said. 'I had my fair share of doubters, and as hard as it is to believe, I still do.'

'You're unconventional, Marc,' she said, 'like Marmite, either they love you or they hate you.'

'Is that a good thing?' I asked.

'It is if you like Marmite.' Her intonation rose at the end of the sentence as if that was meant to mean something more than a comment about breakfast spreads.

'Right,' I mumbled.

There was an awkward pause.

'Are you blushing?' she asked.

'No,' I said.

'Have you got your diary with you?' she said.

'My diary?' I said. 'We've got a wall chart, though it's not very exciting. I mean it doesn't have much in it.'

'Not for the work stuff,' she said, 'I mean I wondered whether you are ever free in the mornings?'

I set my chair back down on four legs.

'In the mornings?' I asked.

Was she asking me out? I grabbed a pen.

'Er… what, after my shift? Yeah, it depends what it is,' I said.

'Don't worry, I'm not about to ask you out on a date,' she said, 'I just wondered whether I could get you in to do an assembly at school.'

'Right,' I said. 'Sure, er, I'd love that. Name a day.'

'Well, Bonfire Night isn't too far away,' she said. 'Could you come in and talk to the school…'

'About checking under their bonfires for hedgehogs?' I said. 'That happens to be my specialist subject.'

*

One, or rather, two of the practice's more colourful clients were sisters. Amber and Amanda were identical twins. Middle-aged and single, the pair lived in an apartment a stone's throw from the surgery. I have never been one to stereotype, but Amber and Amanda were eerily like characters dreamt up in the fantastic imagination of someone like Tim Burton. They were exactly what you would imagine identical twins to be. They were the identical height, they had identical faces, they were dressed identically, their hair was identically coiffed. With Amber and Amanda it was almost if they were not two different people at all, but one, they just took it in turns to talk. And it was almost as if Tim Burton had delivered them scripts in the morning post, and hid himself somewhere just off camera to whisper stage directions into their ears. The cherry on the cake was Amber and Amanda's choice of pet: Siamese.

Dan was trying to teach me a card game when the twins arrived. They rushed in with Bella, one of their three Siamese. The poor cat had collapsed at home with what we suspected was a massive heart attack. I peeked in the top of her carrier and saw the beautiful animal with her warm grey fur lying on the bottom. She didn't move a muscle and her huge almond-shaped eyes were closed. Dan hung back by the sink and watched. He may have been a wisecracker, but it wasn't difficult to read the gravity of the situation. I reached in and felt the left-hand side of her chest to see if I could feel her heart beating. I then checked the femoral artery that runs along the inside of the thigh, one of the best places to feel a cat's pulse. One of the twins clutched the other's hand. Dan rested the sole of his foot against the back wall. I withdrew my hands, and looked at them.

'Amber and Amanda, would it be okay if you wait in the other room for a few minutes?' I said.

They both looked at me with that same look of incomprehension. I held their gaze long enough that they would understand. The news wasn't good. I watched their lips quiver.

'I just want to make a few checks,' I said. 'It's best if I do that here. I'll get Ruth to help you.'

I left the consulting room and walked down the hall to the office where Ruth was certain to be. It was only about 20 or 30 strides to the office but long enough to allow me to snatch a breath from the tension in the other room. It was like someone had opened a window a crack, on a hot muggy day. I hate delivering news like this. Ruth was on the telephone. I walked over and stood behind her. She twisted around when she heard me enter and read in the bad news in my face.

'Sorry, love, can I call you back later?' she said.

Ruth put the phone down.

I sighed. 'There's no vital signs,' I said. 'Could you

take the ladies into the other room and make sure they've got a cup of tea?'

Ruth nodded.

'I'm just gonna do some checks.'

Ruth went to the consulting room and led the twins away. When I walked back into the room, Dan was sitting on a chair, his chin resting in his hands. He opened his mouth to say something then thought better of it.

I picked Bella's limp body out of the carrier and gently laid her on the table. After I laid her down I ran my hands over her tummy. She was bony over her back and had what appeared to be a plump tummy but which was actually a fluid accumulation in the abdomen. This poor cat must have died of sudden heart failure or perhaps Feline Infectious Peritonitis, which is a chronic, wasting disease.

'Has she gone?' asked Dan.

I looked at Fern's impressionable nephew, and nodded.

'There's fluid in her chest. I want to take a sample so we can find out why,' I said.

Failing hearts can't pump enough blood, and allow some of the liquid in the blood to leak into the lungs. It's called pulmonary oedema. When this fluid leaks out and fills the tiny airways in the lungs, it can make breathing extremely difficult and uncomfortable.

Ruth stuck her head around the door. 'Are you alright?' she said.

She was carrying two mugs of tea. I nodded.

'I'll, er, I'll come through in a minute,' I said.

I went over to the supplies cupboard and found a syringe and needle. I inserted the needle into Bella's chest and drew out an amount of fluid. It was clear and watery. I repeated it a few times until I had successfully removed a fair amount of liquid from in and around her lungs.

I peeled off my gloves and threw them into the bin. There's no easy way to tell somebody that their beloved pet has died. People often ask me what to say in that situation. There really isn't a simple answer. Often people feel that when their pet has died they have lost a family member. And it's a sad fact that there is nothing we can say that will make the mourning process any easier. One of the best ways to help someone cope with the loss is to reassure them they are not alone. Offer to help out with arrangements. If their pet is being cremated, perhaps offer to pick up the ashes for them. Or even send them a condolence card.

Dan got up from his seat and started to follow me out.

'Sorry, mate,' I said, 'they'll probably prefer it if there are less of us there.'

Dan nodded. 'Cool,' he said, 'I'll wait here.'

I stood outside the door for a second and took a deep breath, sucking the air in through my nose, holding it there, then blowing it out again. I counted to ten. When I walked into the waiting room, the atmosphere was black. Ruth was sitting beside Amber, with a hand on her knee. Amanda had her handkerchief out, clenched tightly in her hand. None of them looked up. I wandered over and sat myself down in the seat next to Amanda. What do you say? What can you say? The twins looked at me, desperately wanting to hear something good. I followed their eyes as they tightened their lips then looked down at their laps. I leant forward and put a consoling hand on Amanda's shoulder.

'There's no easy way to say this,' I said. I paused. 'We did all we could. I'm so sorry.'

I wished I could have let them know that Bella died peacefully, but with that much fluid in her lungs she would have been in a lot of discomfort. I wished I could have lied and told them it was otherwise, but I couldn't, so there was nothing more to say. We just hung in that moment. A tear rolled down Amber's cheek and dropped into her mug.

'She's gone to a better place,' said Ruth.

The twins nodded.

Suddenly there was a loud noise, a yelp from down the corridor.

'Oh my God!' the voice yelled. 'Oh my God!'

And we all looked up as Dan came screaming into the room. His eyes were wild and his arms were trembling. I raised my eyebrows, in a way that said, Come on, Dan, surely this could wait? What had possessed him? Surely he could read the situation. But Dan had read something he absolutely had to share and he could barely get his words out.

'She's breathing!' he gasped. 'She's breathing!'

Ruth leapt out of her seat, the twins looked completely baffled.

'That's impossible,' I said indignantly.

'Come and see, if you don't believe me,' said Dan.

Normally I would have insisted the twins stay behind in the waiting room while I went to investigate the re-diagnosis of a work experiencer, but this wasn't a normal situation. We hurried into the treatment room and, sure enough, Bella had come round. I couldn't understand it. All the signs of death had been there, yet here she was with her eyes open, slowly stretching out her legs, like she was waking from sleep. Amanda and Amber burst into tears as Ruth stretched forward and stroked her fur. I looked at Dan who was grinning from ear to ear and pacing about excitedly. He couldn't stand still. All I could think was that Bella had been impossibly close to death but removing the fluid from her chest had allowed her to breathe again. She must have been hanging on by the thinnest of threads. I'd never seen anything like it.

I looked at the people standing in the room, witnesses of this miracle and my clunking misdiagnosis. It was marvellous on one hand, but utterly unnerving on the other. I fished about for something to say, but I couldn't come up with anything.

'It's a miracle,' said Ruth, hugging the twins together.

And it was. Their faces were radiant, stretched by two enormous identical smiles. Again, I tried to say something, but my tongue went fat in my mouth.

Amber and Amanda came up to me, each taking hold of my arms.

'We're so glad we came to you,' they said.

I tried to agree with them. I wanted to agree with them, but under it all I was thinking, Why are you so glad you came to me? I've just told you your cat is dead, and it's clearly not.

So instead I beamed a great big smile back as we all bathed in the moment when Bella the Siamese came back from the dead. As the twins stroked Bella's belly, you could hear the tiniest, feeblest purr emanating from inside the cat I had thought had died.

I hate to try to read too much into events, but if there is a moral in Bella's story, then it is this: never believe that you know more than you do, never think you're better than you think you are, and even when you think you've seen everything, always leave room for the unexpected.

I can't say I've witnessed many resurrections. Bella ended up making a relatively full recovery, living quite happily on heart medication for two further years.

There was a big cheesy grin plastered all over Dan's face for the rest of the day. He'd played his part in a minor miracle, and I discovered that behind his joking was a caring soul. He wasn't here on work experience because he had nowhere else to go. He loved people and he loved animals, and what we had just witnessed was a priceless example of what happens when those two worlds collide.

At the end of the shift I make phone calls. Normally when someone asks specifically for me it is something to do with a case I treated either that week or the week before. We are very clear that we only treat emergency cases and refer non-emergencies back to their regular vet. We're a complementary service rather than a replacement. I strained my eyes to make sense of the name Ruth had written down on the piece of paper. I couldn't make it out.

'What's this?' I said.

'What's what?' Ruth replied.

'This number?' I said.

I waved the scrap of paper in the air.

Ruth shrugged.

'I didn't write it,' she said.

'Well there's a scribbled little note here with some-one's telephone number and I have no idea what it says.'

'Pass it here,' said Ruth.

She walked across the room and snatched it out of my hands.

'Paul?' she said. 'Paul Land?'

'Did you write it?' I said.

'No!' Ruth exclaimed. 'I told you I didn't, it must have been Dan.'

'Where is he?'

'He, er, popped out I think,' said Ruth. 'It looks like a Paul Land, yes, I'm pretty sure, though saying that, the "l" of "Paul" does look like an "h" or it could be a "b".'

It didn't matter. I took the paper and dialled the number, and rocked back in my chair. It didn't go through the first time, I just got one of those weird tones that tell you you've dialled the wrong number. I looked at the numbers again and carefully retyped it while Ruth cleared away some things. This time it connected.

'Hi,' I said, 'is that Paul? It's Marc Abraham from the surgery.'

'What time do you call this?' said a familiar voice. 'I telephoned two hours ago.'

'I'm sorry, Paul,' I said, 'this is an emergency surgery and we've been very busy tonight.'

'I'm sure,' he said.

His voice did sound very familiar, but I couldn't place the face. He had a distinctive, a plummy, silver-spoon, Radio 4 broadcaster voice.

There was a pause.

'So how can I help you, Paul?' I said.

'Paul?' he spluttered. 'Paul? Why do you insist on calling me Paul?'

'I'm sorry,' I said, 'it says Paul on the message.'

'Pah,' he said. 'You know very well who I am.'

And then the penny dropped.

'Lord Horncastle!' I said. 'Do forgive me.'

'The stupid neither forgive nor forget; the naive forgive and forget; the wise forgive but do not forget,' he said.

'I'm sorry,' I said.

'It doesn't matter,' Lord Horncastle said, 'it's a quote from a Hungarian psychiatrist. He was a professor in New York.'

I had no idea what he was trying to say.

'I was telephoning, dear boy,' he went on, 'to see if you'd seen the error of your ways.'

'I'm sorry?' I said.

'To see if I could change your mind,' he said.

'About what exactly?' I said.

'Three hundred and fifty pounds to help Ferdinand out of his hole,' he said.

'Are you trying to buy my morals?' I said.

'Oh no,' said Lord Horncastle, 'this isn't a matter for morals. I was just offering to make a generous donation to your good work in return for your assistance.'

'For a testicle implant? Lord Horncastle, I think I made it expressly clear that there is not one ounce of me that would compromise my ethical code so that you can stick a rosette on your jacket. By all means go to your regular vet in a month's time and ask them to see if his balls have descended. End of conversation.'

I'm not sure how much Lord Horncastle heard. The final word was met with that low ringing tone and the disembodied voice of the operator 'the other person has hung up'.

Ruth clunked mugs and spoons loudly in the other room.

'What was that?' she said.

'Well it wasn't Paul,' I said.

At that point Dan bowled into room, bringing an odour of nicotine with him.

'What does this say?' I said pushing the paper under his nose.

His mouth broke into a toothy grin.

'Sorry,' he said, 'when I put the phone down I couldn't remember his exact name.'

'Well what's this then?' I asked.

Dan smirked. 'Posh Lord.'

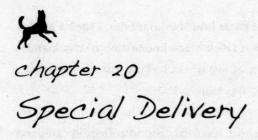

chapter 20
Special Delivery

After the galling episode of the big night out in the summer, I decided to be a bit more proactive in maintaining a more sustainable social life. Looking back at the year, I realised that it had taken me about three or four months for my body clock to completely adjust to antisocial hours, but by the end of it you could say that I had become officially antisocial. It was fortunate, perhaps, that I was single. I'm not sure many relationships could have survived the schedule. Ruth managed somehow, she said it was sometimes a blessing that when she got home she had the house to herself, though most of the time all that meant was that she could Hoover the carpets to Mariah Carey. In order to adjust to my new routine I had gone into hibernation. Which is how that blip in the summertime had happened – I hadn't put the right architecture in place. You can't run your social life like you might run your finances, diligently saving up your credits for a big splurge. And post Beachgate, I was keen to put some architecture in place so I didn't totally lose my social life. The first thing I did was buy a diary

– it was one of those hour-by-hour ones, I took a marker pen and drew a thick black line at two o' clock and a thick black line at five o' clock. That was my three-hour window and it was sacrosanct.

My social calendar revolved around coffees in cafés and coffees in pubs with friends who had the afternoon off or who had sneaked in a late lunch hour. There are hundreds of amazing cafés where I live, classy wine bars and cosy pubs, though the daytime clientele were mums, students or drunks. I was catching up with a friend in a new wine bar that had opened under one of the old arches at the beachfront. A number of new restaurants had sprung up around there, mostly selling fish and seafood. I hadn't seen James for a couple of months. We had met on a scuba diving course. In actual fact, we first met in a flooded quarry in Leicestershire taking our advanced scuba diving course. Forty metres below, in a serious test of the effects of nitrogen narcosis he'd drawn a pair of comedy breasts on my slate instead of the instructed name back-to-front and it pretty much went downhill from there.

'What did you think of the football?' I said.

There was a clunky pause.

'What?' he said. 'Sorry, Marc, you'll have to ask that again. I feel like my head is being pounded by two mountain gorillas with stone paddles.'

SPECIAL DELIVERY

James was nursing a headache. He was permanently hungover.

We caught up as old friends do. He asked me all about the practice and I gave him the warts-and-all rundown. James kept shaking his head and making these sighing sounds.

'It sounds amazing,' he said.

'What does?' I said.

'You know,' he said, 'to be providing such a valuable service. But, boy, I couldn't do the hours. Don't you ever wish you had some time off?'

It was funny looking at James, in his groggy, hungover state. I couldn't remember the last time I had had too much to drink, there simply weren't enough hours in my one day off. Plus there was never anyone to drink with, but I didn't admit to that.

'I'll have a white wine,' James said, as the waitress came past.

'A fizzy water,' I said.

'The hours are a lot,' I said, 'but I do get time to relax. Afternoons for a start, and it's not like I'm always on duty.'

We were sitting at an outside table. It wasn't strictly warm enough to be sitting outside, but we were wrapped up in jackets and coats, and the staff had turned on the patio heater.

'Are you cold?' I asked.

'I'm fine,' said James. 'If I'm honest I could do with the fresh air.'

James wasn't eating but I ordered a chicken quarter, with green beans and dauphinoise potatoes. I never know quite what to order in the afternoon. Strictly it's my breakfast slot but it's also my lunch and I've never been one for brunches. I tend to err on the side of two lunches per day if given the opportunity. James told me about his plan to go travelling in Australia, and how it hadn't worked out with that girl from Essex, but how that was okay because he had got tired of all those Essex girl jokes. The waitress brought us our drinks and a few minutes later out came the food. I was just cutting into a slice of melt-in-your-mouth potato when a lady ran up to our table and pounced.

'There you are!' she said.

The lady was in her seventies. She was wearing a faux-fur coat. She had a pearl set, bright red lipstick, and her hair was coiffured like a Hollywood star.

'Hello,' I said, with a mouthful of chicken, somewhat taken aback. I didn't recognise her from Adam. James's eyes went wide and he leant back in his seat to take it all in. I looked to him for support. He looked back at me, like this was something he believed happened to me every day.

The lady grabbed my arm. 'We saw you walk past our window, Dr Abraham, so I beetled down to find you,' she said. 'And thank God I did!'

A whiff of Chanel blew over us both.

'Prudence has a gone into labour!' she said.

'Who?' I said.

'Pru,' she said. 'Come on, it's an emergency.'

'I'm so sorry, but—'

'Come on,' she said, 'please?'

I looked down at my half-eaten chicken, at the untouched green beans and the creamy potatoes and back up to the elderly lady, tugging on my arm. James beckoned over the waitress.

'Can this be put into a takeaway box?' he said.

A doggy bag may have been more appropriate.

James looked at me with a flicker of excitement in his eyes. 'Come on,' he said, 'let's not hang around. Er, do you mind if I come along?'

Prudence was a Pekinese. The Chinese breed is over 2000 years old. Whilst nowadays the Pekinese are considered toy dogs, they were once believed to have originated from the Buddha himself, and served primarily as a temple dog. This has paved the way for many myths and legends. The most popular story tells how the Pekinese was the offspring of a lion and a marmoset, and to fully enjoy it you have to put to one side everything they taught you in those reproduction videos you watched in your school biology classes. The legend has it that a lion and a marmoset fell in love, so they went to the Buddha for help. He allowed the very big lion to marry the rather small marmoset, but only if he surrendered his height and his might. The Buddha allowed the lion to shrink to the size of the marmoset but keep possession of his lion's heart and character. From this the Pekinese came, or so the story goes. There is another version of the story where the lion instead falls in love with a butterfly, though this seems even more implausible.

The lady who stole us away from our lunch was called Marjorie. Prudence belonged to her neighbour Phyllis. They lived in apartments on different levels in a beautiful Regency building, as close to the beach as you can get. I'd say 'within spitting distance' but Marjorie and Phyllis were not spitting types. As we hurried to Marjorie's apartment we passed conference centres, chain hotels and the independents. There weren't many private residences, but this was the sort of street where property prices went into orbit. We arrived outside their apartment building. From the outside the most striking features were the huge floor-to-ceiling windows behind black wrought-iron balconies that flowed around the side like the levels of the *QE2*. It looked similarly luxurious and similarly iconic. Marjorie's apartment was on the first floor and Phyllis lived above her. They were the best of friends. Both widowed the same year, the 'girls' made a pact that they weren't leaving this world without a fight, and were going to live as full and rich a life as possible. It's actually nice to live on your own, Marjorie told me, when you know you've got someone so close by. They even had a code system. Two rings on the phone meant 'pop down if you fancy'. Two rings in reply meant 'see you in five'.

Marjorie's apartment was stunning. It was the sort of place that needs a baby grand piano if only as a place to display one's silver framed photographs, as the mantelpiece is *so* common. On Marjorie's piano I counted seventeen frames. Most were filled with smiling children, but the large one in the centre had a sepia photograph of her late husband standing by a Spitfire. The front room was stunning. It was the sort of room that wouldn't suit the name 'lounge', it befitted something more grandiose like 'drawing room', the perfect place for daydreaming over a cup of well-brewed tea.

'Marge!' yelled Phyllis from the study. 'Did you find him?'

'Right here!' she called.

James could barely contain himself. He leant in and whispered in my ear, 'I should hang out with you more often.' Marjorie tugged the sleeve of my coat and dragged me towards a pair of concertinered doors. I was marshalled past the balcony from which, Marjorie pointed out, they'd spotted us walking. We were a good few hundreds metres from beachfront promenade.

'You must have incredible eyesight!' I said.

Marjorie pointed towards a pair of binoculars sitting on top of the *Daily Telegraph*, folded to the crossword page, of course. The mind boggled.

Pru was a golden Pekinese. When we walked into the study she was lying on her back in the corner on a poofy cushion that Phyllis had tucked behind her. Phyllis was kneeling in front of her and swivelled right round so she'd see us as soon as we came in the door.

'Oh, Dr Abraham,' she said, 'we're awfully, ever so grateful.' She clasped her hands together, and tilted her head at angle. 'Marjorie and I were going spare. Oh, I say, another dashing gentleman,' she said.

'Hi,' began James, 'I'm—'

'A nurse,' I said, before he put his foot in it. 'We trained at college together.'

'What luck!' she said, and she rose to her feet so we could get a good look at Prudence. For all my joking about the 'Lion and the Marmoset' you had to admit it was a fitting description. She had this beautiful double-thick golden coat that flowed from her broad black face. Her eyes were round and dark, her nose short and wide with these large open nostrils. Prudence was a beautiful dog. But she was in a protracted labour.

Canine labours usually last any time between six and twelve hours. In the first stage, the mother will exhibit nesting behaviour and her body temperature will drop and she'll often appear restless. Stage two labour is characterised by active uterine contractions. In this stage, foetuses are usually expelled within two hours of each other. Prudence had started second stage labour with good, strong contractions but two hours had passed and there was no water bag or puppy. When three hours went by, she'd started crying with each movement. I had always planned to go straight to the surgery after my lunch with James so luckily I had my stethoscope with me in my bag, and my emergency kit in the car. As I moved the cold metal steel of the stethoscope about her tummy I noticed there was part of a puppy presenting, but I couldn't make out what. It wasn't a leg, or a head, maybe it was the neck?

Kneeling on the carpet I had a little flashback. About three years after I qualified, I fancied a break from surgery life so took a short hiatus in my career. I have always been a lover of extreme sports and I was convinced that somewhere in a parallel universe I was a champion snowboarder. Growing up I went on several skiing holidays with my family, and so while I was studying in Edinburgh I made trips up to the Scottish slopes as often as I could. The Cairngorms, Nevis and Glencoe were my escape hatches from the classroom. Three years into professional life, for various reasons, I needed a break. With no job to return to I moved to Val d'Isère and worked a season as a barman. I think it was ten days into my work out there that I let slip what I did back in England, and word soon passed around that I was some kind of Doctor Doolittle. Needless to say, my career break was short-lived. The very next week I helped deliver a litter of Labrador puppies behind a restaurant bar. Fast forward I don't know how many years, and here we were again, albeit in a slightly different set of circumstances. There was no baby grand in the bar in Val d'Isère for a start.

A Caesarean was inevitable. My car was ten minutes walk away, six minutes if we pegged it. I had a quiet word with James and we decided a taxi may be the better option if we could get one immediately. I sent him straight down on to the street while Phyllis went to fetch some towels. With emergency Caesareans, you typically want to get in there as soon as possible. Nevertheless, anything we could do now would save valuable time when we got to the clinic. Before we make an incision the dog's belly is shaved. So I asked them for a razor. Marjorie disappeared off to the bathroom. She was away for some time, you could hear her opening and closing cabinets and turning out the cupboards. Eventually she came running back in, pulling one out of a packet, and juggling a can of shaving foam.

James came tearing back into the room. He was short of breath.

'There's a cab outside,' he said, breaking off to gawp at me kneeling by Prudence with a razor in my hand. Marjorie had wrapped her tightly in a towel to keep her warm and let her know everything would be okay. I quickly finished the shaving, washing the razor with a flourish in a Pyrex jug of warm water that Phyllis had set down.

We got to the practice in record time. I'd put a call into Gloria and asked her to clear the theatre. There was a nurse on hand and pretty much everything we needed. Gloria didn't say a word but gave me one of those sunny smiles that says, *It's all gonna be fine*.

I wasted no time – I was already down to my T-shirt before I was in the front door – got into my scrubs faster than one of Madonna's costume changes and whirred into action. After Pru was happily anaesthetised and her breathing tube inserted, I made a mid-line incision and pulled out the uterine horns. When the uterus was opened I discovered the single puppy with his neck extended over the pelvis and his front legs bent backwards at the shoulders. Puppies cannot be born in this breach position. We removed him, repaired the uterus, and I closed the skin incision with disolvable stitches under the skin so the puppy wouldn't be bothered by the knots when he was nursing. Put like that, it sounds like a quick job, but you have to be incredibly careful and it took around 50 minutes. While I was stitching up, the nurse took on Pru's role of keeping the new puppy breathing and making sure the pup's airways were clear, and James took on my job of keeping the clients amused with quips and jokes. Baby Christopher had entered the world, the most adorable Pekinese puppy with his tiny little legs and his pink snout. Phyllis and Marjorie were gushing. They made a chorus of cooing sounds, and flapped and doted and craned their necks. I walked over to James and leant against the wall in a content and satisfied way.

'Beer?' said James.

I looked at my watch.

There was still an hour to go before I was on duty.

'I could murder a lemonade,' I said, 'plus I've still got half a lunch to finish.'

At that moment Phyllis reached into her handbag and turned her back so I couldn't see, then she shuffled up to me.

'Thank you, Dr Abraham,' she said, 'thank you so much. You've made two little old ladies dottily happy.'

She reached for my hand and pushed in a rolled-up piece of paper. When I looked down there was a 50-pound note there.

'Phyllis,' I said, 'take that back.'

'I interrupted your lunch,' she said, 'you must take your wife out for a dinner.'

'I don't have a wife,' I said.

She looked from me to James and back again with a smirk.

'Heavens, no, it's not like that,' I said.

'I thought for a minute you were Holmes and Dr Watson,' she said.

I tried not to laugh.

'Look, I can't accept this. The surgery will make out a bill,' I said.

'I'll not have it any other way,' she said.

I tried to push it towards her but she kept stepping back. It was no use. She just wouldn't have it.

'All right,' I said, 'you're very naughty. But if you won't take it back, I'll donate it to the local Dogs Trust rescue shelter on behalf of the new baby Christopher… Christopher, Christopher what?'

'Goldstone,' said Phyllis, 'Christopher Goldstone, Christopher Goldstone. Oooh, that does have a lovely ring.'

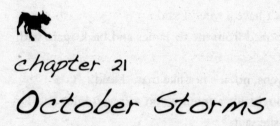

chapter 21
October Storms

Of all the British seasons, autumn's the one I look forward to the most. Over the mild summer, it's like electricity builds in the atmosphere, there's a tingling, unpredictable feeling, and come the first days of autumn it's discharged in all sorts of ways. It shocks the tall deciduous trees and strips them of their leaves, it cranks the thermostat down so your cheeks flush pink and red as you hurry about. Everything about summer is pleasant. It's warm and most people would say it's their favourite time of year. But when the leaves begin to turn, and then a cool wind blows through, there's a feeling that change is on its way, and what's life if it's not about change? I like the brown, reddish colour palette, with the ochre yellows and the oranges, I love the blue of the clear crisp mornings when your words come out as little puffs of steam, I like stodgy puddings and glasses of red wine by a smoky, crackling fire. And I like how the earth makes a crunching sound when you step on it. Summer has a solstice, winter has the longest day, but autumn just seems to roll in whenever it fancies. For most, I suppose, summer ends when the back-to-school adverts return on television, and parents wave their children off to start a new term. But for me, the start of autumn is when I'm walking down the street and a conker drops from a tree and rolls into my path.

I turned the radiators on in my flat on the first day of October. I hadn't deliberately picked a specific day, it was just the first time I felt chilly in the house, and as much as I could hear my mother's voice telling me to think of the heating bills and put another layer on, I was already wearing two T-shirts and a jumper, and I didn't want to look like the Michelin man.

One advantage of working nights in autumn is you get to sleep when the day is warmest, so there's no shivering in bed, or need for a hot water bottle. The obvious drawback is that for most of the time you're awake, you see very little light, and that's enough to send anyone potty.

And then there's the car. Most people's cars can handle the changing seasons, but, unsurprisingly, not the red Cinquecento. I'd put my bag in the back and fished out The Police cassette tape, I was all set to go. But when I turned the key in the ignition the damned engine wouldn't start.

'Did you leave the lights on?' said Ruth.

I was hanging, half-in, half-out of the vehicle with the door open, one foot in the footwell of the car, the other on the pavement, my ancient mobile phone was cradled between my chin and shoulder. I looked like a stressed motorist from a car recovery. I was meant to be in work in 15 minutes, but that looked decidedly unlikely.

'No,' I said a little snappily, 'I drove it back home in the daylight. I wouldn't have had the lights on.'

'You might have knocked them with your knees,' she said.

I pulled an idiotic face, which Ruth, of course, couldn't see.

'What about the radio?' Ruth ventured, desperately trying to think of a helpful suggestion.

'That cuts out when you turn the engine off,' I explained.

Besides, it made no difference, the car wasn't going anywhere fast.

'Are you at work yet?' I said.

'Almost,' she replied, 'a couple of minutes' walk away.'

I shifted the phone to my other shoulder and tried the key in the ignition again. I wiggled it backwards and forwards, as if doing it repeatedly might annoy it into life. But there wasn't so much as a splutter. I've bump-started cars before, but I was parked in a residential bay, sandwiched between a couple of cars, so there was no chance I could get out. I looked up and down the road for a friendly face, to see if I could find someone who might pull in next to me, and dig some jump leads out of the boot.

'Why don't you walk?' said Ruth.

I thought about it for a second. It was tempting. I could get there in fifteen minutes, but the problem was that as much as it was the bane of my life, it was a useful piece of junk – when it worked – and I'd need it if I had to make an emergency call. I was stuck with it, like someone had asked you to babysit, and when you turned up at their house, you found out you were minding Bart Simpson.

'We may need it tonight,' I said, 'I'll call the AA. Can you hold the fort for a bit?'

Ruth laughed.

'Holding-the-fort is my middle name,' she said.

The AA man was a young bloke fresh out of college. He had long shaggy hair and wraparound shades. When I rang they said it could be half an hour, but he turned up within 20 minutes and parked his big yellow van as close as he could, which in my street was about 50 metres behind me. We popped up the bonnet, and he attached the black and red leads of a magic little device that reads the health of a battery. Whatever the state of the battery, there's usually enough residual charge to power the reading device without having to turn it on, so the fact that the screen was blank was not promising. The AA man pulled one of those faces that brings you out in a sweat whenever it's something to do with a car. He tinkered around for a bit longer and I shuffled my feet anxiously on the pavement. He tried the leads in all sorts of configurations and then slowly brought his face up from the engine. The verdict wasn't good. The battery was on its last legs.

'I can charge it up for you,' he said, 'but I couldn't tell you how long it'll last. The problem's that the battery is old and the alternator's not charging properly.'

He ran another health check with a second device that takes a reading, calculates a few things and then spits out a piece of paper that looks like a till receipt. It essentially gives you a pass or a fail. The AA man tore the slip off, folded it in half, and had another go. I guess he didn't have any good news to share. I stood there crossing my fingers, bouncing on the balls of my shoes as he hooked up the leads again and pressed a series of buttons. When the receipt came out, he shook his head, and sighed in that sympathetic way I'd been desperately hoping he wouldn't.

'I think you're going to need to replace both of them,' he said. 'Maybe the alternator would charge a newer battery, I mean, it could just be that that one's overloading it. What I'll do is charge you up, and it should be fine to get you to the garage.'

I thought about what he was saying for a few minutes. The battery had never done this before, and it can't have just magically decided to give up the ghost. I wondered how much I could really get out of it before it kicked the bucket. I mean, these AA guys are professionals; they've got to err on the side of caution.

'Just a thought but how long will a full battery last before it runs out again?' I said.

The young lad looked me in the eyes.

'I mean I've got jump-leads in the back, so...'

He shook his head, and put his hand on my shoulder. I hadn't realised I was that transparent.

'You need to buy a new one.'

The guy stayed longer than he needed. I asked him to fully charge it because the last thing I wanted was the car to stall and have to call them back out again. This was the fifth time the car had let me down in the few months I'd become saddled with it. I had had a new cam belt fitted, new spark plugs, the passenger wing mirror had been smashed off one night by hooligans. The car only cost me £395 to buy, I'd easily spent that again on repairs, labour and wretched parking tickets.

When I pulled into the surgery's car park, the sky was as dark as my mood. A black cloud had rolled over from the South Downs and hung over the city. News and weather reports throughout the day had warned of thunderstorms, and there were flash flood warnings in the *Evening Argus*. And though the rain hadn't started lashing down it was drizzling as if to taunt us. The streets were dark and oddly deserted, as shoppers hurried from store to store. I walked into reception in a stink, about half an hour late. I had the phone numbers of three local garages on a scrap of paper in my pocket that the AA man had kindly written down for me, but I was damned if I was going to call one.

I got changed into scrubs and found a quiet corner to sit and eat a Crunchie – not the most nutritious snack, but I was sulking. Ruth took one look at me and seemingly found a hundred things to do, while Dan stretched out with his feet on an archiving box and watched back-to-back *Superstars of WWF Wrestling* on the television. And then the heavens opened, and I cannot remember the last time it blew so hard.

British weather normally comes in three flavours: fairly mild, mild and extra mild. We don't have the tornados of the American Midwest, the monsoons of India, or the tropical storms of the Caribbean. You'd never find a weather pattern in England that was severe enough to be given its own name – like Mitch, Jeanne or Katrina. But every so often we do get an unusual burst of weather: a heat wave, a heavy fall of snow, or a hurricane. It's nothing compared to weather patterns elsewhere in the world, but the British Isles always goes into meltdown. The newsreaders take it in turns to deliver updates on the impact of the chaos, usually couched in economic terms. When it snows, the councils never have enough salt or grit, travel is disrupted, the schools are closed. The fact is we Brits aren't prepared for anything other than light rain, and the night that we were about to experience couldn't have underlined that fact more.

It was about eight o' clock when the rain started to fall. You could hear it pounding and drumming on the roof like a horde of children stomping about upstairs. A strong wind picked up and drove it in sheets against the windows, lashing and whipping the panes and whistling through the gaps. The animals staying in the hospital overnight were panting and pacing around their quarters. Dan and Ruth went down to check on them, and made sure they were comfortable. I kept an ear out for the practice phone, but it was always quiet on a night like this, as responsible owners made sure their pets were safely inside.

And then, sometime around ten o'clock, we took the call from Mary.

Mary lived in a beautiful old house in a village just north of the city. It was one of those picturesque villages you see in coffee table books about the English countryside, with climbing roses, open garden days and people that look like they come straight out of a Miss Marple mystery. The village had a post office, a church with a spire, a memorial hall and a country pub; every lawn was beautifully manicured and ever other house was thatched, but in the shadow of the thunderstorm, it all took on a faintly creepy demeanour. The pub sign was swinging in its hinges like a creaky door, and the surface of the duck pond was choppy.

We had diverted the phone to mobile and the three of us piled into the Cinquecento. The sky was clapping with thunder, and in the distance we saw forked lightning. The next day we read of the numbers of boats that were damaged as their owners hadn't had time to bring them on to land, we heard radio interviews with stranded commuters and saw pictures of delivery vans battling through floods to reach cut-off villagers. As we drove out to the farm, Ruth anchored herself to the door-handle, Dan bunched his legs up on the back, sitting as low as he could, and I gripped hard on the steering wheel, wondering whether what we were attempting was anything other than foolishness, though when I had put the key in the ignition it had worked first time so I took that as a good omen. My poor little car was buffeted by the winds, batted back and forth across the winding country lanes like a ping-pong ball as the wheels slid and skidded on the waterlogged tarmac.

Mary had telephoned in a state. She was tall and stately looking, an air of privilege about her in her

Barbour jacket and Hunter wellingtons. Once a successful finance director in London, she had taken early
retirement and now lived in an old stone farmhouse with
her two playful Border collies. She'd realised a life-long
dream of living in the country and keeping horses, the
loves of her life. Mary had been brought up in Glouces-
tershire on a farm, and spent every waking minute of her
childhood volunteering at the riding stables, feeding,
grooming, and mucking out the horses, and taking them
on long rides through the Cotswolds with her sister. As
we drove towards her house, seeing her farm up on the
hill reminded me of the sort of place my mother would
always talk about when it came to planning the family
holiday. The cottage shared three acres of land with a
riding stables and countless smaller barns. On a beautiful day, with the windows open and the birds singing it
was a little patch of heaven, but when the thunderstorm
came it looked intimidatingly bleak.

Two great stone pillars stood at the entrance of the
drive with stone eagles wobbling on top, watching for
trespassers. The thunder clapped again above us. As we
drove closer, we began to see the extent of the thunderstorm's damage. The trees were bending and straining in
the wind and, as the gusts coursed about and changed
direction, branches cracked and fell down to ground
only to be whipped up again and carried away like some
sort of torturous game. All three of us were peering out

of the windows. The windscreen wipers were on over-drive and the rain on the roof was deafening. The tree-lined drive was a few hundred metres long and wound all the way from the turn-off up to her house on the top of the hill. We went as far as we could go, and I stopped the car by the obstacle Mary had mentioned on the phone. The winds had ripped a tree clean out of the earth and thrown it across the drive, its huge roots tangled and clodded with earth.

The rain became even more intense.

'We're by the tree,' I shouted into the mobile, cupping the mouthpiece with my hand. When Mary couldn't hear me I turned the windscreen wipers off. It didn't help very much; the rain lashed at us from all sides like we were sitting in a car wash.

'I said we're by the TREE, the fallen tree. T-R-E-E. It doesn't matter. We'll come up to the house.'

I turned to Ruth, and Dan in the back, who looked in no hurry to leave.

'I have no idea if she got any of that, the line was crackly,' I said. 'Ready?'

We took a minute to collect ourselves, and zipped up our anoraks and windcheaters. I fished my woolly hat out of my pocket and pulled it down to my eyes. I had swapped my scrubs for jeans. The North Face jacket I'd found hanging in the surgery belonged to someone smaller than me but it was far less porous than my woollen one. I zipped it up to my chin and did every single popper up. Ruth, in the way only Ruth could, was wearing one of those plastic bag poncho things they sell to tourists and people who visit theme parks.

'You can't wear that,' I said, 'it's blowing a gale.'

But Ruth took no notice of me. She tried to pull a pair of waterproof trousers over her desert boots. The three of us each took a deep breath and heaved opened the car doors into the wind. It was easier on the passenger side, but I had to lean in hard with my shoulder, the doors slamming back in place as we let them go. The thick old trees that lined the path made menacing sounds and tore at their roots like tethered air balloons. We gathered our hoods around our faces, and hurried as quickly as we could up to the house. Ruth banged on the knocker and Mary was waiting on the other side to shepherd us into the warm.

Mary's hands were trembling. She was dressed as if ready to face the elements, but there was no way she was fit to leave the house. Mary told us that her dogs were acting up, but that was an understatement. When she called the emergency line, we kept having to ask her to repeat herself because she was drowned out by the barking and the crashing and tumbling as the dogs tore about the house. Fear of thunderstorms is relatively common amongst collies, but it's rarely this severe. When I was on the phone to Mary, I had asked to describe how they were behaving and she had broke down in floods of tears. Making the decision to venture out in the storm to help her was an easy one.

Mary had bought the farmhouse as a restoration project. The windows were single-glazed, the tiled roof leaked, the old oak doors fitted loosely in their frames. It was a playground for the thunderstorm. Winds rattled the doors like malevolent spirits, shook the windows in their frames and howled down the chimneys. At each thunderclap the collies would tear from one room to the other jumping on tables, overturning chairs, sweeping the mantelpiece clear of vases, photographs and ceramic ornaments. Mary told us they had started trembling and stuck to her like glue and she had tried to comfort them. She stroked their heads and gave them cuddles and got down on their level to whisper reassuring words. But that's when things got worse: instead of being reassured, her words of comfort had set them off on a mad rampage. Babying dogs can have the opposite effect from what the owner intends. You think you're calming them down, but to them it demonstrates they have something to fear. The airline pilot in the storm that acts like it's no big deal is a much better reassurance than a nannying voice on the intercom telling you not to be scared. We suggested Mary could try playing them music, or putting the dogs in their kennels, but the storm was much too loud, and the dogs were out of control. I was concerned that they could seriously harm themselves.

We stood in the hallway for a minute as the collies charged about. One ran in and out of the living room, weaving in between chairs like a skier on the slalom before jumping up on the upright piano. The other slowed when he saw us, broke into a whine, and buried himself in the sofa. I raised an eyebrow at Ruth and nodded towards the kitchen, she understood what I meant.

'Shall I put the kettle on?' asked Ruth. The rain dripped off her poncho and pooled on the stripped wood floor. 'We can leave the boys with the collies,' she said.

Mary made a little nod and led the way. Dan and I went into the living room and shut the door behind us.

Mary had built herself the perfect farmhouse kitchen. In the centre was a huge pine table that could easily seat ten, to the side there was a huge pine dresser with classic blue and white crockery and jugs on display. The floor was paved in brilliant red tiles worn by centuries of farming boots, and the Aga purred away at the end, heating the room with a constant warmth. Then the windows rattled in their frames again like someone had got hold of them. Mary sighed and sat down in a chair.

'I'm so sorry,' she said, 'I'm out of my—'

Mary couldn't finish her sentence, she brought her hand up to her chest and held it like she was in pain. Ruth had her back turned as she filled the kettle from the sink, and opened the cupboards, one by one in search of mugs, spoons, and tea bags. When she turned back round, Mary was hunched over in her seat, her hand in a ball pushed hard to her chest.

'Oh my God,' said Ruth, rushing over from the sink, 'are you all right?'

Mary nodded but took Ruth's hand and squeezed it tight.

'Is there a paper bag about?' she said.

The living room was long but with a low ceiling. A French window led out to the garden outside. The doors should have been covered by a thick curtain but it looked like the dogs had yanked it down; the rail lay on the floor in a bundled mess. Outside tubs and planters lay scattered across the patio, the bigger clumps of mud and dirt that hadn't been picked up by the wind were strewn across the ground. I picked up a squeaky ball and rolled it towards one of dogs and Dan did the same with a Frisbee.

I've worked with similar cases in the past. We're usually called after an incident, when the storm has passed over. In America, where storms are frequent, many owners build thunderstorm desensitisation into their training programmes, but in England, where storms are that much more unusual, we do little to prepare for it. There are two phenomena that can set a dog off – mostly it's loud noises, but it can also be the change in barometric pressure. If the dog is triggered by changes in barometric pressure there really isn't very much you can do. The best thing is to allow them access to a safe bolt-hole like an indoor kennel. You can drape a blanket over the kennel if that helps calm to them down, even throw in a piece of your clothing, and sometimes playing music helps too. If your dog's not a fan of being in the kennel and it makes the situation worse, another thing they often like is to hide in the bathtub. If an animal's fear is triggered by sound, as most dogs are, you can train them with a CD. CDs of thunderstorms are relatively easy to find. If you play it in the house at relatively low levels, the dogs learn to get used to it. You should play with toys and treats while the music's playing but don't cuddle or baby them, associate good activity with the sounds. And gradually over time, increase the volume.

Mary's collies were called Jake and Kettle. They were beautiful black and white two-and-a-half-year-old brothers and Mary had had them since they were tiny pups. Because of the weather they hadn't been exercised much in the day, and since collies are playful animals, they had a lot of pent-up energy which they channelled into nerves. I've seen animals do some crazy things when they're scared, and I was afraid they might do something stupid, like jump through a window. As I put down the toys, Jake knocked over the standard lamp and Kettle burrowed under the sofa. Jake then kicked over a vase, which shattered on impact with the fireplace and sent shards of glass over the tiled hearth. Dan tackled him to the floor and held him tight in his arms until he stopped wriggling.

In these situations there are really only two options, the first is to get them into a safe kennel, the second to use sedatives. I am wary about using drugs. Sometimes drugs can actually heighten fear, rather than reduce it, as when they start setting in and the animal's body stops responding in the way it knows, it can be even more terrifying for the pet. But there are a few cases in which drugs are absolutely necessary to ensure the welfare and safety of the animal.

We sedated the collies, and stayed with them for a while. I checked them for cuts and bruises, but remarkably both seemed to be okay. Dan went on a recce and came back with a broom and a dustpan and brush and he swept up the carnage of the living room, to prevent any possible harm, and to take some of the stress out of the situation. We straightened a few things, reorganised the cushions, and put some classical music on the stereo. I helped Dan put the curtain rail back in place and drew the drapes across the windows. Mary was much calmer when we came into the kitchen. She and Ruth were sitting around the kitchen table, cradling mugs of tea in their hands.

'The collies are fine,' I said. I've given them some sedation to stop them hurting themselves. I don't think they've suffered any scrapes or bruises but it would be good to keep an eye on them.'

At that moment there was another loud clap of thunder and the horses screamed.

chapter 22
Heartbreak on the Hill

Mary had been in no state to get the horses out of the field and into the safety of the stables. She'd noted the skies were darkening and watched the weather change, but she couldn't have known what strength of a storm was brewing, and how severe its effects. Mary had had an early evening meeting with a charity she volunteered with in town, they were arranging a local fundraising event for the old people's home, and by the time she'd got back home the winds had picked up and were blowing strong. An empty grain sack landed on the grille of her car and slipped up the windscreen, it gave her quite a shock, and when Mary opened the front door, the dogs were doing laps in the hall, and they rounded the corner and knocked her over. The next thing Mary heard was an almighty crash and the sound of plates smashing. Lying on the welcome mat, the front door slammed shut behind her. Mary propped herself up against the wall. She sat herself calmly on the carpet and put a hand up to her chest and tried to steady her breathing, but the dogs didn't calm down and the winds didn't stop. In the past she'd had panic attacks that lasted ten or fifteen minutes; this time they came one after the other, forming a cycle that lasted several hours.

If she had hoped she could just sit still and ride out the storm, Mary was sadly mistaken. The storm clouds were moving slowly, building and darkening exponentially, like a snowball growing in size as it rolls down a hill. And off in the distance there was thunder, hard to make out at first, a soft, low rumble like a hungry stomach, but the rumble grew into a thud and the thud grew into a crash and the crash sounded as if the sky was being rent apart. Given her emotional state, perhaps Mary should have called for an ambulance for herself, but with the horses running scared and the dogs charging round the house, it was us who took the call. She was paralysed by the thought of the poor horses out there in the field.

Mary was staring at the surface of the long pine kitchen table. She was drawing her finger around and around in tight circles. I looked at Ruth, who had a hand on her shoulder. And then Mary's lips moved without her looking up.

'The horses,' she said, 'we need to put them in the stables.'

There was a sudden loud crack as another fork of lightning struck the earth and almost immediately the sky rumbled, loud and deafening. It seemed that the storm was right above us. I could hear the horses whinny in terror out in the fields. Mary pushed back her chair, which squealed on the tiled floor. She leant on the table top to help get herself upright, and began to zip up her coat.

'There are three of them in the field,' she said, 'between the four of us we can get them all in.'

'Are they tied up?' I asked.

I had visions of the horses tied to metal posts or railings or even to trees, with lightning striking around them. Lightning always targets tall objects and metal things; electricity tries to find the path of least electrical resistance. Horrible images forced themselves into my brain. But Mary shook her head – they hadn't been tethered. It was both a good and a bad thing. Had they been tied and spaced out so they could see each other, they may be a little calmer and would be easier to gather, but thank God they weren't tied to a lone tree or a pole.

I put my hand on Mary's. 'Are you sure you want to bring them in?' I asked.

There's long-running debate in the States about whether a horse is better off in a barn than in the open air during a storm. Inside seems safer, away from the lightning, the trees and open spaces. In high winds debris, building materials and even farm equipment might be thrown into the air. But some horses get spooked in confined spaces and that can only make things worse, there's plenty of material around for them to injure themselves on. Besides, there's always a chance that lightning would strike the barn and cause a fire, which means that the horses would be trapped inside. There's no right answer. There are countless stories of horses in the open fields being struck by lightning or hit by debris but similarly thousands of tales of horses surviving ninety-mile winds without so much as a scratch. It's really up to the person who knows their horses best.

'They live in the stables,' said Mary. 'They're used to it. I'm very careful not to leave them out at night.'

She pulled an anguished face, we could all see what she thinking, but she was at the mercy of her medical condition. There was another blinding flash of lightning and a loud clap of thunder.

'Wait,' Ruth said, her face pushed up to the window, 'not now, it's right above us. We should wait for the lightning to subside before we start rounding them up.'

Ruth walked over from the window and grabbed me by the elbow to make sure she had my agreement and one by one we settled back down into our chairs.

'Another tea?' said Ruth.

Every year lightning strikes kill tens if not hundreds of people in the UK and thousands across the world. Because we don't have them that often in England, we can be quite blasé about it. Whenever there is a storm the father of a friend of mine goes outside and sits in a metal chair in his back garden to watch 'nature's firework display'. I think he gets some pleasure from defying Mother Nature but his family keep telling him it's only a matter of time before he's hit. And you don't even need to be directly hit, just being in the dispersion path can provide enough current to stun the heart. It's incredibly dangerous to be out in a lightning storm, which is why Ruth wanted us to choose our moment.

We huddled in the kitchen and waited. Mary drummed the table with her fingers, Dan and I watched the storm rage outside. Ruth was right to call us to wait, the lightning had been right above us. You can tell how far a storm is by timing the gap between the lightning and the thunderclap. Sound travels about a mile every five seconds so if you count 'one thousand one, one thousand two, one thousand three' and so on, you can estimate how far away it is. The next flash came in about thirty seconds, and this time the sound gap was longer, the storm was passing over and moving on. We waited for five more minutes before leaving the house.

The horses were running around an open paddock surrounded on all sides by high wooden fences. The storm may have been moving on, but the winds were still blowing strong. There was a small clump of the trees at the back of the paddock that looked so bunched together it was if they were practising safety in numbers. The horses would run over and shelter under them but the sound of branches cracking or snapping and the high winds sending pieces of debris in the air would trigger them off again into a wild run. They'd do a couple of laps and then fly back. The horses were worked up and panicked, throwing their heads about, moving errati- cally, this way and that, like they couldn't make up their minds where they wanted to be heading. One of the horses, a beautiful dark brown stallion named Captain, kept running to the tallest oak tree that stood alone in the middle of the pasture. He would wait there for a little bit, flicking his head about, then dart off to find somewhere else to shelter.

We hadn't talked about how we were going to go about rounding them up, but Mary was an experienced horse-handler and she took the lead, buoyed by the support she had from the three of us. We trudged up the fence and one by one climbed over. The plan was to move as a group and round up one horse at a time. There was no need to whistle or shout a name. As soon as the dapple-grey mare saw us she trotted over from the small clump of trees straight to Mary. Mary grabbed her halter and kissed her nose.

'That was easy,' said Ruth.

'Can you take her?' she said to Dan. 'She's called Pinto.'

Dan gripped the halter tight and gently stroked her head.

The wind was still shaking the trees and snapping branches though the thunder was quietening down. A shadow moved out of the clump of trees and trotted over to where we were standing, picking up speed when he saw Mary and Pinto by the fence. Felix was a beautiful black Arabian horse and he ran straight over to Mary, slowing only when he got close enough to nuzzle her shoulder with his nose. Ruth took hold of his halter and she and Dan held the two horses together, stroking their noses with the flats of hands and telling them they were all right. But the brown stallion wouldn't come.

'Captain!' Mary shouted.

She put her hands on her hips and bellowed across the field. 'Captain! CAPTAIN!'

I joined in. He flicked his head round. We knew he'd heard us. Mary put her fingers in her mouth and let out a high-pitched whistle.

'Captain!' I yelled.

But he didn't come.

Mary edged forwards a little. The horse was tearing around the field, darting this way and that, rocking forwards then pulling back as if he was caught in car headlights.

'Captain!'

We stood there and waited, hoping he would turn around, but he seemed to pick up pace. He darted to the lone oak tree again, stopped for a second and then tore off to the clump of trees at the far end of the fence.

'Captain!'

And then it happened. Mary whistled. I had my arms raised, waving at him. He stopped and turned around.

'That's right,' I said, 'come on.'

Captain took a few steps and came a bit a closer. Pinto and Felix tugged on their halters as if they were joining in the effort to beckon him home, and Captain started to trot towards us, but suddenly there was an almighty clap of thunder, and he reared up on his back legs with his front hooves in the air. For some reason he changed course, and galloped faster and faster and faster towards the fence nearest the tree-lined drive where we had come in. He went past the lone oak tree standing in the centre of the field, picking up speed as he went, and as he neared the perimeter he took off, leaving the ground. Captain tried to clear the high wooden fence, and got his front legs over, but just his front legs. The beautiful brown stallion came down hard on the fence post, and my heart and my stomach were in my mouth. He let out a cry and Mary collapsed to the ground.

We didn't go back to the surgery that night. We took a few calls on the mobile but there was nothing that couldn't wait till the morning. We did everything we possibly could to save Captain's life, but the post had gone deep, and even with the local villagers to help, we couldn't lift him off it, however much we tried. I called for back-up from two or three large animal vets, but the injuries he had sustained were just too much. In the morning we had to hire a crane to help. Mary knelt in the mud beside him and buried her face into his neck. Dan and Ruth led the other two horses into the stables and made sure they were safe and comfortable.

We were all in shock and floods of tears; it was the single most tragic incident I think I have ever witnessed, and Ruth, Dan and I didn't really speak about it afterwards. I'm pretty sure that I cried more that night than at any other point in my career. The predicament was just so helpless. My brain was swimming with questions. I ran through hundreds of different scenarios. What if we had done this, or what if we hadn't done that? Who's to know what would have happened to Captain had we not been out there to round him up? But had we not been out there when he jumped the fence, his passing would have been much more to bear. We were able to limit his pain and in the end we helped him on his way so his last breaths were as quiet and as peaceful as they could have been. But that night was by far the most traumatic thing I have ever experienced

Mary, unfairly, will always blame herself. For months afterwards she put the horses in the stables every time she left home. And you'll never hear the weatherman in her house. She turns off the radio when the weather forecast is broadcast and changes stations when it comes on the news. Ruth and Mary formed a close bond in the weeks that followed. Ruth voluntarily took it upon herself to help her through the grieving process and to make sure that Mary didn't carry the blame alone. Ruth helped train the collies with the thunderstorm CDs, and over the weeks, Mary found it within her to move forward. Three months later there was a new arrival at the farm – Blue, a sweet gentle mare that she adopted from Horse Rescue. And these days, if you visit the farmhouse it's not rare to hear the laughter of children. Mary offers the use of her farm to a local equine-assisted therapy organisation that works with children and young people. In that way she helps other people overcome all sorts of issues through their interaction with her horses, the loves of her life.

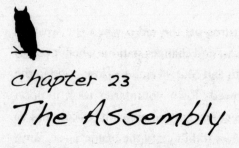

chapter 23
The Assembly

It was a Thursday morning and we'd finished the shift, but the night, or rather the day, was far from over. There was that rare thing on the wall calendar, an entry, and for the morning too. In big black letters I had scrawled 'Assembly'. I was going to visit Fern's school.

'How do I look?' I asked Ruth.

She looked me up and down.

'You look great,' she said sarcastically.

I scowled.

'Well, what am I meant to say?' Ruth said. 'You're wearing scrubs, you wear them every day, I mean, what should I comment on, your shoes?'

She had a point.

I was meeting Fern in the road outside the school. I had suggested we met in the car park, but she said she didn't want to give the game away. She'd been telling the children that they had a very special visitor and they were excited. We met up at the back of the school, or 'behind the bike sheds', as Fern put it, and I was to be smuggled in through the delivery doors to the kitchen. Fern was waiting for me in her car and stepped out when I pulled up. She gave me a hug and a kiss on the cheek that was a little close to my lips.

'I feel weird about this surprise,' I said. 'They're going to be crushingly disappointed when *I* step out on stage.' I opened the back door and took out my winter coat. It was bitterly cold. My breath made clouds in the air as I zipped my coat up over my uniform. 'They're probably expecting a footballer from the Albion or something.'

Fern laughed. 'Well, I can't speak for the rest of them, but my class are Man United fans,' she said.

I looked at her with a smirk.

'And you?' she asked.

'What?' I answered.

'What's your favourite football team?' she said.

I smiled. 'My favourite football team?'

She nodded.

'Arsenal.'

'Great,' she said with a smile on her face.

I laughed.

'Do you find it difficult to switch out of classroom mode?' I said.

'Not really,' she replied.

She turned to enter the school grounds. I caught her by the arm.

'You just asked me what my favourite football team was like I was an eight-year-old boy in your class, and I said Arsenal, and you said great. That was sweet.'

Fern glowered at me.

'No, it's funny,' I said, 'I mean it's sweet.'

Her eyes narrowed. 'Marc, don't you think I might have asked because I like football, or were you assuming that I'm not into football because I'm a girl?' she said.

'What's your team then?'

'Norwich,' she said. 'Spurs beat us in the cup, and if you'd said Tottenham I would have thanked you for your time, marched you straight back to the car, and explained to the children that the speaker had to cancel today because he came down with scurvy.'

'Okay,' I said.

'What do you say?' said Fern.

'Sorry,' I said. 'Now I really feel like an eight-year-old.'

'Wipe that smirk off your face,' she said.

The primary school that Fern taught at was only a short drive from the practice. She explained to me that there were approximately 400 pupils aged between three and eleven, and they were divided into 15 classes each named after a different bird, from starlings to kestrels and penguins. If I was there, I think I'd be a dodo. Before school, Fern told me, the kids would meet up in their classrooms and catch up about what happened on *Top Gear* the night before or regale their classmates with their stories of successes on the Nintendo. At 8.25 on the dot a buzzer would sound and one by one the classes were called to the assembly hall. To ensure they had everyone's full attention, and to make sure it was fair, classes were called at random.

'Magpies and Sparrows,' the tannoy announced, with a little flourish of birdsong.

The head teacher was a bird enthusiast and had a series of different calls that he would blow after each announcement, mostly, I think, for his own amusement.

Fern and I sat at the front of the hall on a raised stage but hidden by a curtain. The whole place smelt faintly of Dettol, and I watched a cleaner tackle a puddle of vomit with a bag of sawdust. It was an assault on the senses and spookily reminiscent of my own days in education. Then came a sound like a polite herd of elephants that had been told to walk not run. Another buzzer sounded and the Larks and the Night Owls were summoned. I peeked out from behind the curtain. There was a scrum to sit at the front. As soon as the children got through the door, the 'walk don't run' rule went out the window as they waddled, jostled, skid and slid as quickly as they could to nab the best patches of floor space on which to park their bottoms.

Within five or six minutes the room was full. I'd visited classes before, but I had never spoken to an assembly and I wasn't prepared for the sound of a hall brimming with children. The only thing I can equate it to is the noise of a leisure centre swimming pool on a Bank Holiday Monday. There were giggles, shrieks and titters, pushes and pulls, loud voices, shrill voices, clapping and singing, but the second the buzzer sounded again, the room fell silent in an instant.

Fern turned to me and smiled. 'You'll be great,' she said.

And she pushed aside the curtain and stepped onto the stage.

'Good morning, school,' she said in a loud, teacherly voice.

'Good morning, Miss Gilmore,' they chimed back in unison.

'We have a very special guest today. Before I introduce him, does anyone have any idea who it might be?'

A forest of arms went up.

'Before I ask one of you, I'm going to give you a clue. Think about what event is coming up this weekend, and ask yourself what professional person might be coming in to give some very important advice.'

The arms dropped. Four hundred children's heads clunking and whirring, them one by one the arms went up again.

'I'm going to take three guesses,' she said, 'Jane.'

A little girl in the third row back looked to the left and to the right and realised that Miss Gilmore did mean her.

'A witch,' she said.

There was an intake of breath.

'Not a witch,' said Miss Gilmore, 'Halloween was last week.'

There was a collective sigh of relief.

Miss Gilmore pointed to another child.

'A pumpkin,' said Tommy.

The whole hall burst into fits of laughter. Tommy looked pretty pleased with himself, and collected his pats on the back with a grin.

'Sensible answers, please,' said Miss Gilmore.

She pointed to a little girl sitting quietly on the front row. She was easily dwarfed by everyone else, but stuck up her hand as high as it would go.

'Lucy,' she said, 'who do you think it might be?'

All eyes turned to Lucy. She looked coyly at the floor and wound her finger into her skirt. Then in the softest of tones, she said: 'I've forgotten.'

Miss Gilmore shook her head.

'All right,' she said, 'well, I'll let him introduce himself then. Put your hands together for Dr Abraham.'

I got up from my plastic chair, came out from behind the curtain and walked to the centre of the stage.

The whole room room gasped. Four hundred pairs of eyes were staring at me in my greeny-blue scrubs.

'Good morning, everyone,' I said.

'Good morning, Dr Abraham,' they sing-songed back.

It was a little more subdued than I had expected, but perhaps I should have been quicker to reassure them that I wasn't a dentist. Dentists wear a similar uniform and I am sure half of them were terrified to open their mouths.

'What day is Saturday?' I asked.

'Guy Fawkes Day,' said a smart-looking boy in the front.

'That's right, and what's so good about fireworks day?' I said.

I picked a sweet-looking girl.

'Burning stuff!' she said.

They certainly were cute.

I trotted out the usual talk of checking for hedge-hogs in the garden when they got home and then it came to matter of pets and fireworks. Every child in the room had something to say on the matter. They hopped up and down on the floor like they were sitting on an anthill. I have never met a child who doesn't have a question or a story about animals and I was starting to relax into it. The trick, I had figured out from speak-ing to individual classes, was to ask questions, make it interactive. I wasn't sure if that would work in an assembly but it seemed to. Fern was beaming away at the sides.

'Okay,' I said, 'now this is the really serious bit. Are you all listening? I want you to turn to the person on your left and right and say, "Listen, this is important!"'

The kids did as I said and the hall floor bubbled with excitement.

'Okay,' I said, 'who here has a pet?'

Across the room hands popped up like mushrooms.

'All of those with your hands up, does anyone know what you should do with your pets on Bonfire Night? I'll give you a clue, fireworks can be very loud!'

Three rows back a boy's arm shot into the air and he groaned like he was in pain. I could have picked any one but this kid looked like he would pass out if I didn't choose him.

'Okay,' I said, pointing to the boy. 'What's your name?'

His eyes went wide. 'Scott,' he said.

Scott was about seven or eight with a wild crop of blond hair.

'What pets do you have?' I said.

'I have a cat called Oscar,' he said, 'he's a white one.'

'A white one?' I said. 'Very nice. So, Scott, what should you do with Oscar on Bonfire Night?'

'That's easy,' said Scott. 'Take him to a bonfire.'

The hall broke into laughter again. Scott looked quite put out. He stuck out his bottom lip.

'No,' I said. 'Why would you take Oscar to the bonfire?'

'Because it's really, really cold outside,' he said, 'and cats are warm. I am warm, Oscar is warm and a fire is warm. Together we'll all be really warm, we won't even need to put on our coats.'

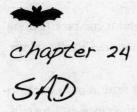

chapter 24

SAD

Dan had done his last day with us a couple of weeks before and since he'd left, work had been getting noticeably longer and harder. In November the days are brutally short and the nights painfully long. When your schedule sees you in bed by nine in the morning and up again at four or five, it is possible to go through an entire week seeing maybe two or three hours of sunlight. I moved to Brighton because I loved the sun, and the beach, I'm an outdoorsy guy. Yet there were days in that first winter when I thought I may as well have been working in an underground bunker in Coventry or Derby or somewhere equally drab.

I casually mentioned this on the telephone to my mother one night and instantly lived to regret it. I had just been thinking how relieved I was that the flurry of concerned 'tiredness at work' emails and helpful suggestions had dried up and then I go and drop a clanger like that.

Mum went quiet on the phone.

'What?' I said. 'Oh no, don't you do this...'

'Do what?' she said, innocently.

'Mum, please don't worry about me or email me links or text me questions. It's nothing. Really, Mum, it's fine,' I said.

'But it could be serious. I've read about people in dark countries and how it affects their moods,' she said.

'I'm not down,' I said. 'I'm happy.'

'Okay,' she said, 'but—'

'No buts, Mum, I'm fine. Please don't worry.'

There was a pause.

'Do you promise you won't worry?' I asked.

'Yes,' she said, grudgingly.

A couple of days later I was woken by the doorbell. It was the postman with a parcel. I couldn't quite believe my eyes when I opened the package. A bumper pack of vitamin D tablets and a clipping from a magazine article about SAD in Nordic countries. The journalist pointed out that the suicide rate in Iceland is much smaller than he would expect and how, in fact, SAD levels are very low indeed, not because of genetics, he suggested, but because of the large amount of fish the Icelandics eat, 225 pounds per person per year as opposed to about 50 pounds in the United States. There was a Post-it note clipped to the news-paper cutting:

I didn't pack you any tuna because I figured you had good enough access to fish where you are. Keep drinking lots of fluids.

Much love, Mum.

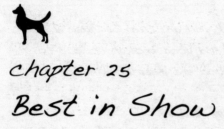

chapter 25
Best in Show

I love dog shows. Most shows take place in the earlier parts of the year, but where I live, there's always a charity dog show in the autumn in one of the villages that surround Brighton. Because there aren't many shows at this time of year it gets pretty busy and since it's a large fundraising event it's a huge amount of fun, especially if, like me, you have a weak spot for lemon drizzle cake.

The show always takes place in the recreation ground. With the help of some sticks, perimeter tape and a handful of traffic cones, the cricket pitch is magically transformed into a serious-looking dog show-ring. The small brick village hall (rebuilt and extended with Lottery money) is transformed into the dog show nerve centre, with cakes set out on fold-out tables, coffee granules lining the bottom of Polystyrene cups, and steaming urns of boiling water. A team of elderly women potter around with cloths and paper towels to mop up the spillages of the over-excited children who are chasing toy dogs, gun dogs and hounds around the room and bashing into the legs of tables, chairs and vicars. The old ladies tut, and natter amongst themselves that they wouldn't have been allowed to do that in their day, and they weren't given half the things these kids got, they got a lump of coal and an orange for Christmas and were grateful for it. At that point a child will slam into the table which is holding the squash and knock over a jug of blackcurrant, turning the floor into an sticky ice rink. This happens every year.

There are two types of dog shows, the serious, official, pedigree ones and the anyone-can-enter novelty fun ones. This show was a weird mixture of the two. I don't think it would be unkind to say that it was ostensibly a fun village dog show that fancied itself on the Crufts circuit. I happened to know the man in charge, and he was nothing if not ambitious. He had contacted a cohort of local celebrities to attend, and been largely disappointed with their responses. The previous year he managed to secure one of the Gladiators to open the show and was a bit put out when he turned up. It seems that he was a little chubbier these days and wasn't wearing his Lycra unitard. The ex-Gladiator explained that since the television series had not screened for many years and he couldn't get into his costume any more, he'd eBayed it to raise money to buy a motorbike. Over coffee, the organiser told me that 'looking at his jowls' the publicity photographs the Gladiator was signing had to be ten years old.

The organiser was called Derek. He was a short, wiry man, with boundless energy. From the minute he woke to minute he went to bed he was always on the move. He was a proponent of standing-up meetings, an American business idea that says you get a lot more done if, instead of sitting down around a table, you held your meetings standing in a circle. It sounds crazy but I have no doubts that this works; it would be difficult to fall asleep in a PowerPoint presentation. But where would you put the plate of biscuits? After a local newsreader dropped out, Derek had asked if I wouldn't mind standing in as a judge. I've judged events a few times before and dutifully obliged.

I arrived a little late for my briefing; it seemed a little overkill to hold it two hours early. I found a space for the Cinquecento and hurried over to four people standing in a ring on the field. Derek was in a blue blazer, and wore a Panama hat that he'd ordered from an advert in a Saturday newspaper.

'Marc,' said Derek, shaking his head, 'where have you been?'

'Saving lives,' I said, jokingly.

Derek wasn't really listening, he was looking at the face of his watch.

'You're eleven minutes late. We had to start, in four minutes I need to brief the tombola team.'

Derek took me to the boot of his car where he made me try on a selection of hats and blazers. None of the blazers seemed to fit. They were either too long or too short.

One of them fitted like a glove, until you got to the sleeves, which stopped quite a distance from my wrists. Derek yanked them down as they far as they would go.

'You did bring a white shirt, didn't you, Marc?' he said.

'Yes,' I said, nodding. It wasn't ironed though.

'There'll be an inch of white cuff,' he said, shaking his head, 'so keep your arms by your sides as much as possible, any sudden, jerky movement will push them back.'

'Okay,' I said.

'It's not your fault. I had everyone's dimensions weeks ago, but so-and-so pulled out at the eleventh hour. I'm just pleased I'd ordered spares. Now, you'll have to find one of the other judges and get them to talk you through the briefing. It's all in the email I sent you, but I do find it helps to go through it with someone else. Follow the laminated signs to the judges' enclosure; they're affixed to every other tree.'

I raised my eyebrows.

'It's in the mothers and toddlers room. There's an ironing board set up already,' he said. He looked me up and down. 'I'm guessing you'll need it?'

The dog show was one continuous show that fell into two parts. There were all the usual categories you'd expect from a serious show and the categories you'd expect at a fun one. At the head of the list were the big ones, the gun-dog group, the pastoral group, the working group, the utility group, the terrier group and the hound group. The toy group bridged the gap into the more lighter classes – any variety puppy, dog with the waggiest tail, prettiest bitch, most appealing eyes, most handsome dog, and then my category, the special category – best rescue dog. Rescue dogs are the reason for the whole day, all the proceeds from the event are given to the local animal shelter.

Within an hour the car park was packed. There were hundreds of people, and countless numbers of the four-legged kind. The sound was truly deafening. In my experience it doesn't seem to matter how serious the dog show is, you always get serious show-ers, and they're incredibly competitive. Today was no different. Everywhere you looked, you saw estate car boots open, there were owners with their brushes and combs, they had more stuff with them than my mother ever took with her when we were youngsters. Mum would just pack some hankies and a packet of Fisherman's Friend.

The day started early and ran to a tight schedule. There was initially a lot to do, shirt ironing, judge meeting, reading through print-outs, official photos, chats with the volunteers, but when Derek picked up a megaphone and called five minutes to the grand opening, all the pre-activities stopped, and everyone convened around the cricket pitch. There were hundreds of spectators. Most of them had brought their own camping chairs and warm rugs to drape over their knees. I found myself walking around with a can of Coke to keep me awake. I checked the time on my phone. I'd been up for fifteen hours already.

In the middle of the field was another fold-up table, filled with 15 or 20 gold trophies and numerous coloured rosettes. To the side was a little stepladder, whose purpose soon became clear as Derek climbed up three steps to give himself a little pulpit and with a pop and a crackle the megaphone turned on.

'Will all competitors for the gun-dog category make their way to the registration tables.'

The crowd broke into applause. We were off.

It was a brisk, chilly morning, but the sun was dazzling. It was the sort of light that means you have to squint or use your hand like a visor. After five or so minutes of doing this, I decided the best course of action was to fetch my sunglasses from the car. It was as I nipped back to get them, that I bumped into a German shepherd called Ferdinand.

Lord Horncastle was dressed like a true country squire. He was on his knees on a *Telegraph* supplement, protecting his red corduroy trousers from the squidgy mud behind the Land Rover, wielding a grooming brush. He was wearing a soft flat cap, smart brown brogues, an immaculate tweed jacket, blue striped shirt and a magnificent lemon yellow tie. Ferdinand eyed me suspiciously as his owner brushed and fluffed his chest fur. As luck would have it, our cars were parked almost side-by-side, we had happened to park in the same row, there was no way we weren't going to have some interaction.

'Good heavens,' I exclaimed, 'look who it is.'

Lord Horncastle briefly looked up from his grooming.

'What are you doing here,' he asked me with a sneer, 'shouldn't you be in bed?'

'I'm judging today,' I said deliciously, 'and you?'

Lord Horncastle went white as a sheet.

'You. You're judging?' he said. 'You mean you are judging the show?'

I nodded.

'But...what?...right..er...'

'Don't worry yourself,' I said. 'You'll be pleased to hear that I'm not judging your class.'

I opened my car door, and rifled in the door pockets for my sunglasses. In the door mirror I watched him fish around in his pockets, pull out the order of the day and scan the category listings, I assume, for the names of the judges.

'Ah, rescue dogs. I love rescue dogs,' he blurted out. 'Damn fine work those charities do.'

My Ray-Bans were in the glove compartment.

'What did you say?' I said, turning round, and putting the glasses on my forehead.

'Rescue dog charities,' he said, 'a damn fine business.'

I humoured him with a nod and started off back towards the pitch. When I drew parallel to his car, I stalled.

'Your class is soon,' I said. 'I would normally wish you luck, but I don't suppose you've left much up to chance.'

I watched Lord Horncastle for his reaction. Rumbled. He didn't know what to say.

'Good luck, anyway,' I said, walking on. 'I'd best be off.'

'Dr Abraham!' he called. 'Wait up!'

Lord Horncastle jogged over. He came beside me so we were eyeball-to-eyeball.

'I've been thinking for some time I'd like to give a donation to the work of the rescue shelter.'

I smiled.

'That's great,' I said, 'I'll let them know. Good luck today.'

As I took my place in the crowd the first category was in full swing. It was the gun dogs, and on the cricket pitch a retriever was being led around in a circle as a cocker spaniel waited his turn. Derek was over by the stepladder. He picked up his megaphone again.

'Will all pastoral competitors and exhibitors please make their way to the registration table.'

I'd been tracking Lord Horncastle and Ferdinand, they had waited by the side gates and, as they now made their way through the barricades, the posh Lord looked decidedly sheepish. Ferdinand, for the record, looked typically magnificent. The judging falls into two sections, first the exhibitor stands still with their dog while the judge makes an inspection, then the dog gaits – moves at a steady pace – so his movement can be assessed. Derek picked up the megaphone and called hush for the awarding of the gun dogs, but my eyes were on Lord Horncastle, handing over the paperwork, and getting his show number. There weren't many in the pastoral category, a couple of collies, a corgi, another German shepherd and Ferdinand. They lined up and one by one they were brought forward for inspection. Each inspection took a couple of minutes. Lord Horncastle pulled out his handkerchief from his sleeve and mopped his brow. This was going to be interesting. At that precise moment I felt a tug on my sleeve. It was Derek with a clipboard.

'Just to give you a rundown of your category. Now you know how these things work, I suppose?' he said.

'Yes,' I said, somewhat distracted by the activity in the pastoral section. The judge was inspecting the corgi.

'Well,' said Derek, 'just so we're clear, the prize isn't necessarily awarded to the best showed dog, we always try to give a platform to their stories. Marc, are you listening?'

'Yes,' I said, 'a platform for their stories.'

'Right,' he said, 'you've got four in the category: a three-legged poodle, a cancer-survivor, a Staffie-cross that was found in a wheelie bin, and a triple-road accident escapee.'

He handed me a clear plastic folder with their stories in.

'We asked each owner to write five hundred words. Have a read before you get out there, Marc,' he said. 'Marc!'

Ferdinand was up.

Derek tapped me on the shoulder. 'Give me some confidence I've made the right choice,' he said.

'With what?' I said.

'With you,' said Derek.

The judge started at Ferdinand's head.

'Right you are,' I said.

The judge inspected the teeth, his back and tail.

At that point the judge crouched down to inspect Ferdinand's hind legs. There was no reason for him to feel the testicles, and, you know, it is amazing these days what miracles surgeons can perform, I'm sure they looked very realistic. Lord Horncastle looked away. He daren't look in the judge's eyes.

'I mean, how do you begin to decide which animal deserves the award when you've got a shortlist like that,' I said, only half paying attention. 'I'm sorry, Derek, I need to watch this.'

And then it happened. The judge paused. He had another look. He shook his head. Then he stood up straight and asked Horncastle a question.

'What are you looking at?' asked Derek.

'Just watch,' I said.

Lord Horncastle leant in and said something, and the judge shook his head again. He beckoned one of the other judges to come over for a second opinion. They talked for a moment while the other exhibitors stared, and murmured amongst themselves. Lord Horncastle stood there like a lemon. The judging was halted for a couple of minutes but it felt like an eternity. Lord Horncastle was getting restless, he couldn't stand still. The crowd began to stir, no one knew what was going on. Finally the judge came forward and the adjudicator went back to her seat. Ferdinand was disqualified.

'Would you excuse me a minute?' I said.

Lord Horncastle's face filled up with red and he glared in my direction. He didn't wait to hear any more.

'Come on!' he grunted, tugging Ferdinand's lead.

The crowd got to their feet.

'Ferdinand!' he called. Lord Horncastle gave his dog a little push, and the pair hurried out of the arena as quickly as they could, breaking into a trot at the gate in the direction of the car park. I followed them at a distance. Lord Horncastle was in a right old stink, ranting at the heavens, kicking the dirt. He went straight over to his Land Rover and got Ferdinand straight in the boot. I waited till he was in the driving seat until I came up to the window.

'What happened?' I said. 'I thought you had it sewn up.'

Lord Horncastle wouldn't look me in the eye.

It turns out he thought it was in the bag as well, but Mother Nature had other plans. Lord Horncastle had managed to persuade another vet to give his magnificent dog testicle implants. All to win a rosette. It should have all been fine, but what Lord Horncastle had failed to notice was that since he'd put the artificial ones in, Ferdinand's real testicles had decided it was time to come down, and when it came to showtime the rather over-endowed Ferdinand was disqualified. Horncastle's show career ended with a wheel-spin out of the car park and a raised middle finger standing in the air.

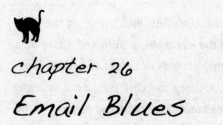

chapter 26
Email Blues

From: Mum
Date: Thursday, 1 December, 9:31 am
Subject: Music

Marc, I know it's pointless sending you this but
Mandy was cutting my hair the other day and she
said when she's feeling blue she listens to music to
reset her mood. She says why don't you try listening
to songs that are about the different seasons, like
'Four Seasons in One Day' by Crowded Houses. Do
you know Crowded Houses?

Sending you my love, Mum x

EMAIL BLUES

From: Marc
Date: Thursday, 1 December, 03:42 pm
Subject: Re: Music

Hi Mum, thanks. Listening to music really helps.
I haven't heard of Crowded Houses but I have been
listening to this band called Travis. They have an
excellent song called 'Why Does it Always Rain
on Me?'

Love you, Marc.

chapter 27

Christmas is Coming

I'm Jewish, so when I was growing up, Christmas was never quite as much of a riot as it was for everyone else in my school. My family isn't a particularly Orthodox, so my parents tried to include as many of the normal Christmas traditions into our own 'holiday'. We had turkey made the Delia Smith way and all the trimmings, we had paper crowns and crackers, we had Christmas television and family arguments in the afternoon, we just did it all on Boxing Day, so there wasn't any confusion.

I love the Christmas build-up. I used to swear it got earlier and earlier each year, but this year it seemed to take some time to spring up on me. Perhaps it was the hours I was working. One of the downsides of working night shifts is when to hold the Christmas party. It was the first week of December and we were in the middle of a cold snap. The roads were clear as I drove into work and the rain was lashing down. The little wipers of the Cinquecento were breaking their backs to swish the water left and right. Michael Buble was on the radio. A lady ran across the road with shopping bags filled with toys and games. I let out a long sigh. Hello, Father Christmas, it's nice to have you back.

Ruth was up to her festive best. She had a Christmas tree earring in one ear and a red parrot one in the other. Apparently she spent her last Christmas in Peru and she wanted to be transported straight back when she caught her reflection in the bathroom mirror.

'You should wear a paper crown,' she said, 'cover up your baldness.'

'I'm not bald,' I retorted, 'this is purposefully shaved.'

'Purposefully shaved?' she snorted. 'That's funny.'

Ruth wound a length of tinsel around in her hair.

'Take that off,' I said.

'Why?' she said.

'Because you never know what we might have coming in today; I don't want you talking to a distressed owner dressed up like a Christmas tree.'

Ruth didn't reply, but she unwound the decorations from her hair and tied them to the standard lamp in the waiting room.

'Scrooge!' she grumbled under her breath.

Things ramp up at Christmas. In the run up to the festive season, when there's turkey, presents and parties on the brain, pets are often the last things we think about. It's understandable, but we always try to remind owners of a few basic things, like anchoring the Christmas tree so it doesn't topple over, covering up electric cords and flashing fairy lights, keeping holly and mistletoe out of reach, and the one that lots of owners forget: don't hang chocolate decorations from the tree.

June was something of a supergran. She'd taken early retirement to help her daughter out with her two sons. I have never seen two children with so much energy; I suspected that they were half human and half Tasmanian devil. It was as though their mother kept them in a cupboard and force-fed them Sunny Delight, releasing them occasionally to wreak havoc on the world. Everywhere they went they left a trail of destruction behind them. They weren't evil, they were just, well, boys. And I'm a big fan of kids using their imaginations, but I genuinely believe these tykes would have plotted and carried out a successful military coup had they been given the time and the appropriate arsenal.

June looked after the boys after school while her daughter finished her shift at the BP garage. She usually worked from 10.30 in the morning to seven o'clock at night, manning the cash register. She'd pick the boys up on the way home, and nine evenings out of ten June would have a meal ready for her, unless she was going out for a night with the girls at the ladies' bowling league.

That night, June had popped out to Tesco to pick up a few essentials, and when she got back, the boys were worked up into a frenzy. June was weighed down with heavy shopping bags, two or three in each hand. The boys waited by the door to pounce. As soon as they heard the key in the lock and saw the handle go, they grabbed her by the arms and pulled her towards the kitchen.

'Hey!' said June, taken aback. 'STOP it!'

They were tugging on her hard.

'STOP IT! What's got into you?'

'Poppy's died!' the boys said.

June's heart stopped beating.

Poppy was the name of June's golden retriever, and the love of her life. When Alf, June's husband passed away, the family bought her the most beautiful puppy you could picture. Full of life and with boundless energy, Poppy was so much more than a pet, and the boys totally adored her. She was always doing something daft, she'd chew everything she could get her paws on, remote control cars, mobile phones, DVDs, even slippers.

'She's under the Christmas tree,' they said. 'Come quick.'

Leaving the front door wide open, June dumped her carrier bags and ran in, setting milk and eggs spilling everywhere. The living room was fairly small and the Christmas tree was ginormous. If you're going to decorate the house you may as well go all out. It was one of those trees that was so big you had to saw the top off to fit it in, and though it had only been indoors a few days it was already dropping needles. Under the giant tree, where the presents soon would be, lay Poppy, stretched out, motionless, with a big swollen belly.

'Poppy!'

The boys stood over by the door and looked like they were about to cry. June crouched down by her side and stroked her belly. The branches above her were totally bare. Poppy was lying on a bed of pine needles. There were foil wrappers littering the carpet and only a handful chocolates still hanging on the higher branches.

'She eated the chocolates, didn't she, Gran?' the boys said.

June turned around, and slowly nodded her head.

Poor Poppy had munched her way through 13 chocolate Santas in their coloured foil wrapping.

'We saw her licking her lips for ages,' the boys said, 'and then she started to cry.'

It was high drama when they arrived at the practice. Poppy couldn't walk, her back legs buckled when she tried. With help from a neighbour they had carried the four-stone girl to the back seat of the car, and drove straight over, without even telephoning. One of the boys sat in the back, and whispered encouragement into her ear, the other rode up in the front, wrapping his head around the seat backs to watch. We heard the commotion before we saw them. June came bursting in. 'Can someone help me with my dog?'

We dropped what we were doing.

Ruth and I followed her out to her car. The boys were squabbling in the back. Poppy was crying. June's phone went. I caught snatches of the conversation: 'I'm at the vet's...Poppy's eaten chocolates...the boys are here...no, they didn't do anything...chocolate...it's poisonous...'

I took Poppy in my arms and carried her across the tarmac and into the practice.

'How many do you think she's eaten?' I asked.

June pulled a face.

'There were twenty in the pack, I think,' she said.

Chocolate may seem a trivial thing, but to dogs it can be deadly. As humans, we just think it'll harm the waistline and rot our teeth. To dogs, chocolate is equally morish, but potentially lethal. The toxicity of chocolate for dogs is due to its theobromine content, a chemical in the cocoa bean that is similar to caffeine. And if you think posh chocolates might be better, think again. Those Green and Black's dark chocolate bars may be organic and tasty but they're stuffed full of theobromine. Because chocolate looks so harmless, as opposed to something like rat poison, it's easy to overlook it as a threat. That's how it has become one of the most common poisonings to occur to pets, especially around Christmas and Easter.

It would be tempting to point the finger at the two boys but symptoms like these usually present between six and twelve hours after ingestion, so it was likely Poppy just fancied something sweet to nibble on after her lunch. You'll usually witness some degree of acute abdominal pain followed by explosive diarrhoea, but in the most severe cases there could be fits or even a one-way coma. I've heard of fatalities from dogs eating a large amount of chocolate and going untreated. A vet in my last practice witnessed two such cases. In both instances it took little more than a handful of chocolates.

Deaths amongst quite large dogs left untreated are not in any way uncommon.

'Has she vomited?' I asked.

'I don't think so,' said June. She looked at the boys. They shook their head.

'Tremors or spasm?' I said.

'No.'

I listened to her lungs, the breathing was quick and irregular. It was a good sign that Poppy wasn't fitting; a convulsing dog would need to be immediately admitted to intensive care for heavy sedation. My main concern was to get as much of the poison out of her stomach and give her something to slow the absorption of the toxic substances into her intestines.

We gave her an apomorphine injection to induce vomiting and then put her on a drip. It wasn't long before poor Poppy repeatedly vomited up various puddles of partially chewed and digested chocolate all over the hurridly put down old newspapers, with its sweet distinctive smell. She was lucky June brought her in before the symptoms worsened. Poppy was going to be fine. She made a full recovery.

'Well done for bringing her in so quickly,' said Ruth.

'Don't thank me,' said June, 'thank the boys. They were the ones who spotted something was up.'

I looked around the room.

'Where are the boys, out of interest?' I said.

It didn't remain a mystery for long.

There was laughter coming from reception, and not an adult laugh. It was the laugh of two pre-pubescent hyenas. June went charging out. Ruth and I exchanged glances. We counted to ten. Then the air filled with the blood-curdling scream of a grandmother coming to the end of her rope.

'KYLE!' she yelled, 'GET OUT OF THE FILING CABINET!'

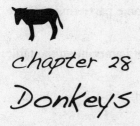

chapter 28
Donkeys

'Ta-da,' she said, 'the Christmas party.'

Ruth had brought some Lambrini and I had a bag of sausage rolls and Hula Hoops from Sainsbury's. We were standing in the kitchen looking at our modest little haul. It was like we were schoolkids plotting a midnight feast.

'Would you like some coffee cake?' said Gloria, taking pity on our rather humble little celebration. 'In fact, I may have some Jaffa Cakes left, if you promise not to eat all of them.'

She cleared away some mugs and reached to the back of the cupboard where a Tupperware box was hidden.

'Things go walkabout in this place, doesn't matter if you write your name on it, put up signs.' Gloria gestured to a printed sign Blu-tacked to the cupboard door. It read: 'Thieves Will Have Their Hands Cut Off!'

'That's pretty punchy,' I said.

'It works in Iran,' she said, 'and some parts of Swansea.'

She tore open the top of the container.

'Ooh,' she said. 'I've got some party rings. There you go, that's my contribution.'

Gloria looked at the bottle of Lambrini on the table and frowned.

'Who brought that?' she said.

I pointed at Ruth.

'Don't worry,' I said, 'we'll only have one glass.'

'I'm not worried about that,' said Gloria, 'I know you'll only have one glass. Have you had it before? It tastes worse than my mam's ginger wine, and there was never anything remotely ginger or wine about that, I can tell you.'

'Damn!' I said. 'I haven't called Fern.'

Ruth and Gloria made knowing eyes.

'Another date?' said Gloria. 'Lucky girl.'

I rummaged about in my bag for my phone.

'We haven't been on a date,' I said.

'What was drinks last week then?' said Ruth.

'A planning meeting,' I said.

Gloria gave me an almighty wink.

'A planning meeting?' she said. 'Is that what they call it nowadays?'

I looked up from my bag. 'We were planning the school nativity play.'

Ruth nearly choked. 'You're helping with the school nativity play? I didn't know you were a hit on the stage, Marc. Are you playing Baby Jesus or the donkey?'

Gloria was beside herself.

'I think both of you are forgetting that I'm quite well connected in the animal world and if Fern wants Joseph to ride in on a donkey, then I'm going to get her a donkey,' I said.

'You are joking aren't you, Marc?' said Gloria.

Ruth looked at Gloria and Gloria looked at Ruth.

Ruth went first. 'Let me get this straight. You, Marc Abraham, are helping supply an actual real-life donkey to a primary school production of a nativity play?'

'You promised her an actual donkey?' said Gloria.

I nodded.

'You're out of your mind,' she said. 'You're crazy, Marc. You can't promise her a donkey.'

'I did,' I said.

'Who's going to "lend" you a donkey?' said Ruth.

'I've got it all planned out,' I replied, 'and before you ask, you can't have tickets. They're for parents only, and they're all sold out. Now pass me the Hula Hoops, let's get this party started.'

(For the record, Gloria was absolutely correct. I defy anyone to drink a full glass of Lambrini and enjoy it.)

chapter 29
A Fox in the Cold

It felt like a classic case of déjà vu. Ruth and I were in the Cinquecento, the night shift was over, and we had one last stop to make. We crossed the same traffic lights, waited at the same junctions and turned down the same roads into the same quiet residential street, where unbeknownst to all but a few, Brighton's foremost husband-and-wife animal rescue double act lived. We pulled up outside and parked behind their little blue Metro in the drive. The one with the large seagull sticker on the rear window, the emblem of the football club, and the bird that was more than a recurring theme in their lives. We stood outside on the front door rubbing our hands together to keep them warm.

'Look at me,' I said to Ruth. 'You may be about to see some gerbils. So no cutesy noises, no mushy stuff, no goo-goo-ga-ga nonsense, all right?'

Ruth nodded.

'I'm serious,' I said, 'we have a reputation of professionalism to uphold.'

Fleur opened the door. She had two baby gerbils in her hands.

When Ruth caught sight of the newborns, the baby gerbil faces peeking out of her hand, she completely and utterly melted.

'Awwwwwwww,' she squealed, 'wook at their wittle noses.'

Fleur was beaming. I wasn't.

'Ruth!' I said.

'I can't help it,' she said. 'I'd been mentally preparing myself to see *one* gerbil all the way here in the car, and then there's *two* of the little bundles. *Two*. Aren't they the most perfect wittle thwings?'

'Yes, they are. Aren't you?' said Fleur, ever so gently stroking their heads with the tips of her fingers.

I stood on the doorstep, shaking my head.

We weren't here for the gerbils this time. Roger had received a late-night phone call from a lady down the road with an injured fox in her garden. A lot of injuries to wild animals occur around this time of year, either road traffic accidents in country lanes when drivers aren't paying attention, or problems with litter. In the party season households create more waste. Home-owners may not think twice before they throw out huge numbers of bottles or cans, boxes or polystyrene that can be hazardous to curious animals, and in towns streets are filled with pint glasses and discarded beer cans.

Roger was in the kitchen having Marmite on toast. The counters were full of crumbs, and the knife was lying on the side with a buttery trail smeared behind it. The morning radio show was in full swing, which was still a little disorientating for us, as we'd just finished our 'day', and were ready to go bed.

'Good morning, Marc,' he said, between mouthfuls, 'and you must be the famous Ruth.'

We shook hands. Roger was a big man, which surprised me when I met him, probably because Fleur was so small. He brushed some crumbs off his mouth with the back of his hand.

'Thanks for coming out. The lady's house is just down the road. I didn't want to move it, in case it's worse than it looks,' he said.

'It's a fox?' I said.

Roger carried his plate to the bin and scraped the leftover crusts with the side of his knife.

'A young cub. Can't be much more than a year old. It's not a pretty sight. It looks like she's been hit in the eye by a firework,' he said. 'Makes you want to cry.'

It was a short walk to the neighbour's house. Roger and Fleur grabbed their coats and a torch and the four of us walked along the pavement of the quiet cul-de-sac like a crack SAS choir of carol singers doing an early morning reconnaissance mission.

Their neighbour (Julie), was an animal lover. Though feeding foxes is generally frowned upon, she couldn't help but leave out scraps of food and water for the fox family who walked along her fence and stopped off in her garden. They'd visit in the early evening and the little cubs played in the grass, scrapping and howling and tumbling. But Julie noticed that something was different this week, and when she came out in the morning to take away their dishes, there was an orange ear peeking out of a cardboard box by the tool shed, an orange ear that belonged to a little fox cub, shivering wet in the rain.

Julie was waiting for us at the front door. She was tall and cheery, the sort of person who looks right at you when they talk. She wore a big baggy sweatshirt with Daffy Duck on it, grey and softened through hundreds of washes and tumbles. Julie was a single mum. She had a son called Donny on the severe end of the autistic spectrum whose best friend was their cat Charlie. Charlie was more than a pet, he was Donny's best friend; when Donny wouldn't talk to Julie, he'd talk through Charlie. Julie said she spent hours every week sitting outside Donny's door, just eavesdropping on the conversations he had with their cat. It was often the only way she could find out how her son was really doing, whether he was being bullied again at school and what other kids had said to him. Donny was upstairs playing computer games when we got there. Julie led us into the hallway and called up the stairs.

'The vet's here, Donny,' she said, 'I'm just taking them out to the shed.'

She lingered at the stairs for a minute with her hand on the railing.

'I doubt he'll come down,' she said to us in a hushed voice, 'he doesn't do well with strangers.'

I followed Julie's big hazel eyes up the stairway and imagined what it would be like to have a son you loved more than anything else in the world, but was a constant struggle to connect with.

'What games does he play?' I asked her.

'Oh, war ones, mainly,' she said. 'He plays other people around the world on the Internet. He can't see them, you see, so it's easier. You can pretend to be anyone you want.'

We walked through the living room past two empty bowls of cereal and kids' cartoons on television and out the double doors into the garden. There was a short paved patio that turned into a narrow strip of grass that stretched a long way, and running around the perimeter was a high panel fence. Julie wasn't the gardening type, it seemed like she dabbled but only did the bare minimum. The grass went from well-kept lawn to knee-high in the space of 15 metres. At the top end by the house were pots of perennial plants but as the garden sloped down the flowerbeds became increasingly over-grown and brambles crawled everywhere. Right at the bottom of the garden was a tumbledown shed and a pile of branches.

'I'm sorry it's such a mess,' said Julie, stepping over a shattered flowerpot. 'I know this is going to sound weird, but I do it deliberately.'

It is hard to see anything in the early morning light and we only had one torch. We walked in single file with Julie leading the way and Ruth and I behind. Roger and Fleur smiled as we steered them around an old wheel barrow that was somewhat concealed by high grasses. Julie held the torch and occasionally the light beam flashed against things, and we saw stuff we hadn't noticed before. There were feeders in every conceivable place, bird houses nailed to trees, and pine cones hang-ing from tree branches that Julie told me she'd spread with peanut butter then rolled in bird seed, a slap-up feast if you've got a beak.

'I was brought up in the country, you see, and I like to be near the wild. Cities give me the shivers. I'm sorry. I keep the garden like this deliberately so it's a bit wild, so we get all sorts of visitors. Every day I wake up and hope there'll be a deer, but it hasn't happened yet.'

I totally knew what she meant. I grew up in the suburbs. A place caught in the crossfire between city-life and the countryside; I know where I'd rather have been.

We walked on a bit further, and then the pace slowed. Julie told us to be quiet as we approached the tumble-down shed. We were looking for the cub. We stopped a couple of metres away and Ruth and Fleur dropped back so we wouldn't overwhelm her.

I couldn't see her at first. It was hard to pick out much.

'Over there,' Julie whispered, gesturing towards the gap between the shed and the fence. There was an old cardboard box. It was a big, kitchen appliance size box. It must have been outside for a while; the cardboard was wet and soggy and there was a hole torn, or perhaps bitten, in the side. Roger and I crept up and as we edged closer we were able to look. At the bottom of the box, curled up like a shrimp, was the terrified fox cub. Julie had brought down a blanket and she had wrapped herself inside it with only her face peeking out. The fur on her head was matted and wet. In the opening of the box were two dishes, one filled with cat food, the other with a single piece of white bread, and the tiniest puddle of milk. Roger bent down and moved slowly towards it, the fox cub turned her head, and I saw for the first time the state of her right eye. When I was growing up, a boy in my class spent two weeks in hospital after a fireworks accident. Children had been throwing them in the street and he looked over the fence to see what was going on and caught one in his eye. He suffered permanent eye damage. His mother campaigned for years to have fire-works banned, but every year there are still thousands of incidents.

We were now a few feet away. Usually you wouldn't be able to catch a fox but this one was so sick it just lay there. The golden rule is not to approach an injured wild animal like a fox, they have needle-sharp teeth and may bite. Roger was wearing protective gloves. He sent me round the other side of the box and we gradually closed in.

'It's okay,' Roger repeated under his breath, 'it's okay.'

The cub was crying. They were quiet, mournful cries. A fox cub usually cries when it's hungry, trying to command their parents to feed them, but this cub had been like this for hours, her parents were nowhere to be seen. I peered in through the side of the box, the whole right side of her head was inflamed and her eyelid was lacerated. The socket was swollen and infected, but her cornea was ruptured, with the iris prolapsing out through the hole. Roger whispered my name and I reached up to see his hands stretching out and reaching towards the cub. We had tranquillisers with us, but it didn't look as if we'd need them. Sometimes when you see footage of young wild animals it's hard to see them as anything other than something from the world of Beatrix Potter, but foxes should be thought of in the same way as cats; they can leap up and bite at any moment especially when scared. Their claws are fiercely sharp. Roger told me later that he usually catches a fox with a net, or cubs with a blanket or a thick coat. Darkness is reassuring for the fox, as it is a nocturnal animal it helps them feel safe.

Roger scooped up the cub in a bundle of blanket, and slipped on a muzzle like he'd done it a hundred times, and with the cub in his arms, we turned quickly and walked back towards the house. As we got the patio Donny's face appeared at the window and pushed up against the glass.

At the back of Fleur and Roger's house were two long buildings. One was a converted garage, the other a long shed. I say shed, but it was so much more than that, it was a permanent wooden room with windows and a carpet and inside there was space to house and rehabilitate injured animals. It was bright and clean, there was a sink over by the window, and a long treatment table. He had latex gloves and swabs and ointments, and along the floor by the wall was a line of carriers and cages. Roger wasn't a veterinarian though, he did only basic rehabilitation and the scale of the cub's condition was far worse than he could treat, the cub would need to go to hospital for surgery. Usually, as an emergency vet, I'd refer anything, but I was well aware that Roger worked out of the kindness of his heart, and had to foot the huge medical bills himself. Roger carried the cub over and laid her on the treatment table. He, Ruth and me huddled around the blanketed bundle (Julie was on the school run).

'Thanks for your help,' said Roger. 'I'm sorry to have called you out. I just thought it was smart to have you along in case something else was wrong. I'll drive her to the hospital.'

He stood over the fox cub, you could see him counting the cost of the hospital treatment. With Christmas coming up, family budgets are always tight, and this family was far larger than mummy and daddy and two point four children. I looked at my watch, it was almost nine o'clock, we were officially off duty.

I beckoned Ruth over and whispered in her ear, 'Are you free for the next couple of hours?'

Her eyes lit up and her lips parted into a smile.

'Let's do it. I'll get the box of tricks,' she said, and she disappeared off to the car.

We thought 'Holly' would be a good name for her, because we found her in the cold. The procedure took a couple of hours. We had to remove her eye, and stitch her eyelids together. We put her on a course of antibiotics, antinflammatories, and gave her a buster collar to wear to stop her scratching the wound. It's always sad to have to lose an eye, but she'll manage just fine with one and be a perfectly active vixen. I've performed the operation for several dogs. Even totally blind dogs manage very well in familiar surroundings and they're never bothered by only having one eye, once it's healed.

Roger was over the moon.

'You guys,' he said, 'are angels. Let me get a picture of you two with Holly for the website.'

We crouched down by the treatment table where Holly was still under as Roger rummaged in a box in the corner for his digital camera. Ruth put her arm around me.

'This has been one of the best years of my life,' she said.

I didn't know quite what to say.

'Say cheese!' said Roger. 'After three.'

Just as he said it Ruth tipped back her head and let out the most almighty yawn. You know how infectious yawns are. Ruth managed to compose herself by the time Roger pressed the button, but for ever now, frozen in time and preserved on the world wide web is a photograph of the two of us: Ruth, beaming from ear to ear, and me with a great big mouth cave, as if I was catching flies.

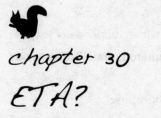

chapter 30
ETA?

The first thing I thought was that I was being abducted by an alien spacecraft. I couldn't see a ring of light around my bed or feel any tractor beams, but I could hear this strange pulsing alien warp sound. It was like something out of *The X Files*. I lay in my bed, not moving a muscle, and waited for them suck me up into the sky. It was then that I realised that it was my stupid phone.

'Hello!' I said, sleepily. I'd perfected my isn't-it-obvious-I'm-sleeping-I-work-nights-don't-you-know voice. I rubbed my eyes.

'Hello?' I said again.

'Darling,' said the voice, 'I thought you weren't going to pick up.'

I rolled my bleary eyes.

'Well I did, Mum,' I said, 'what time is it?'

I rolled over and looked at the face of my alarm clock.

'It's twelve fifteen!' I said. 'Why would you call at twelve fifteen?'

'Dad wanted to know your ETA,' she said.

I took a deep breath.

'My what?' I said.

'Your ETA, your estimated time of arrival,' said Mum.

I was rather blunt in the morning.

'For what?'

'For Boxing Day,' she said. 'It's just there's a Christmas Art Fair in Stanmore and we wondered whether we should all go. Your sister's gang are all coming.'

'Boxing Day is over a week away,' I said.

'It pays to plan ahead, darling,' she said.

'But not at twelve fifteen.'

'No need to be snappy, Marc,' she said, 'I was just calling about your ETA.'

'I don't know… lunchtime?' I said.

'It sounds like someone got out of the wrong side of the bed this morning,' Mum said. 'I'll tell Dad you'll be here for lunch.'

'I haven't *got out* of bed, I've only just gone to sleep,' I said.

'Then roll over and get some sleep, or you'll still be in this mood tomorrow.'

I did. It didn't work.

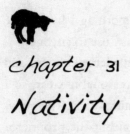

chapter 31

Nativity

I'm in two minds about school nativity plays. Is it a cute bunch of kids joyously re-enacting the Christmas story, or a disastrous mess of squabbles, tears, stage fright, bad music and even more suspect costumes? I may have been brought up Jewish, but I didn't attend a Jewish school, and having a loud singing voice (more loud than tuneful) I was always roped into the performance. I think it would have been weird for the Jewish boy to play one of the starring roles in the birth of Christ, so perhaps on those grounds I was usually first pick for the farmyard chorus. I played a sheep, a snowflake, and quite a convincing donkey, if I say so myself. And now it had come full circle.

The donkey sanctuary was in Sussex, not far from where I lived in Brighton. The team had very kindly agreed to help, but I had to get there early – early being some ungodly time like 10.30, which for anyone else would be leisurely, but for me meant about an hour and a half's sleep. I'd bought one of those magic coffee machines that makes espressos with a little pod that looked like a flying saucer. That morning I had to use three of those pods before I was any use to anyone.

The trusty Cinquecento didn't let me down, and the roads after rush hour were reasonably clear, so I pulled in to the sanctuary ten minutes early. The nativity play was not till the afternoon but the proprietor of the sanctuary was keen that we had time to talk things through and make sure everything was okay. We'd already discussed how the school was really keen for a child to lead the donkey out, with another child riding on its back. After a short confab it was decided that to have a child lead a donkey with another child on the back was asking for trouble, and she suggested we could do one or the other, either have a child leading the donkey out with a handler waiting just offstage, or a handler would lead the donkey out with Mary on its back. I passed the ruling to Fern who thought that a child in a dressing gown being led onto the stage on the back of a live donkey would be more than enough. She was beside herself with excitement.

My phone beeped in my pocket. It was a text message from Fern. 'HAVE U GOT IT YET? X', it read. 'JUST PICKING IT UP NOW. IT'S GOING TO BE A RIOT' I replied.

How true.

The sanctuary wasn't just for donkeys, they would

take any unwanted animals. There were Shetland ponies, sheep and pigs; each animal there had a story.

There were a handful of cars in the car park, but no one obviously waiting. I sat on my bonnet for a bit and waited for someone to pop out from behind a horsebox, but everyone must have been busy at work. I pulled a scrap of paper from my pocket on which I'd scribbled the proprietor's name. Polly. I dialled the number below it. Straight through to voicemail. I started to walk back to my car when I heard my name being yelled across the yard. I spun round to see a woman with a platinum-blonde head of hair hanging out of an open window.

'I'm over here,' she said.

Polly dressed like a fading Hollywood queen. She had an air of Joan Collins about her. Her hair was big and bouffy and perfectly coiffed, there were pearl studs in her ears, and she wasn't shy with the make-up. The reason she hadn't come out to greet me became abundantly clear when I opened the door of the office. The office was a prefab building, like one of those offices you find at a building site. Polly was sitting by her desktop computer with her leg resting on a cushion, she had it raised up on the desk under a bag of frozen peas. A black puffa jacket hung on the back of her chair.

'I can't believe how silly I am sometimes,' she said. 'I slipped on the ice. I was lucky I managed to break my fall. Look.'

She pulled back the sleeve of her sweatshirt and showed me a grazed, swollen arm.

'Oh dear,' I said. 'Does it hurt?'

'A bit,' she said, 'and today of all days.'

The ramifications hit me. *Oh no*, I thought to myself, *she's not going to tell me what I think she is, is she?* My mind went to all the worst-case scenarios. I suddenly pictured myself dressed as the back end of a donkey costume, with some old sweaty PE teacher at the front.

'Don't worry, the donkey's fine, I just don't think I'll be the one leading him on,' she said.

I breathed a sigh of relief. 'Thank goodness. I thought you were about to say we couldn't do it. Who's going to lead him out?'

Polly looked at me. 'Well, you'll be okay with it, won't you?' she said, 'I can guide you from the sides.'

'Me?' I laughed nervously, hoping she was joking.

'Of course,' she said, 'who else is there?'

I looked outside at the horsebox, and the ponies in the field. I nodded sheepishly. I put my hand in my pocket and felt the mobile phone. It was too late to back out now.

'Will you pass me my crutches?' she said.

Polly hobbled her way down the path to the donkey field. They had five, she told me, some of them were quite rowdy but a couple of them would 'do the job'. This didn't instil me with much confidence. There was

Chloe, the mother figure. She was the pacifier, Polly told me. If any of them got a bit rowdy, Chloe would quiet them down. There was Treacle, who was a little shy. He used to give rides at funfairs so you'd think he'd be good with children but he was terrified of everything, particularly cars. There was Bodger, who was just about the wildest donkey they'd ever had. With a bit of training, he'd calmed down, but with those hooves, on a school stage, you wouldn't want the risk. As we leaned over the fence and sized up these powerful, sort-of tamed animals, it dawned on me that what we were doing was absolutely nuts, and when Polly, leaning on her crutches, started talking about kicking and dangerous hooves I started to feel physically sick.

'Do you have a lot of schools coming to visit?' I asked.

Polly thought about it before she answered.

'We did,' she said, 'way back when. Not so much these days. All the health and safety stuff nonsense. Ooh, what about Rapunzel?'

Polly made this clicking sound with her mouth and Rapunzel came trotting over.

'She's six years old, she used to be tied up most of the day near a pub. All day, every day, she did nothing but put up with drunk parents and their kids. She's got a real heart of gold, this one. Come here, Rapunzel,' she said.

Rapunzel was a beautiful donkey, with a soft fair coat hence her name. She sidled up to Polly and snuffled the flat of her hand.

'She'll be perfect,' Polly said.

'She's good with kids?' I asked.

'An angel,' said Polly, 'a darling. She's the tamest we've got.'

Polly leant over and tugged my sleeve.

'You'll be fine,' she said, 'I'll be just offstage with a bag of sugar lumps. Right, let's get a move on.'

'Hi, Fern, it's me. I'm just phoning to let you know we're on our way.'

Fern's mobile went straight to voicemail so I figured that she must be in class.

My hand was shaking. I clenched the steering wheel hard in my hands till my knuckles went white. It was one of the most nerve-racking drives of my life. Stop-start, stop-start, stop-start. I was more nervy than when I took my driving test. 'Take it slowly, slowly, SLOWLY,' I kept repeating under my breath as we hared around the country bends.

We travelled in convoy. Polly, Rapunzel and the stable assistant in the horsebox leading the way, with me a safe distance behind. It was Polly's suggestion that they went up front, so I could make sure that nobody crashed into her. A safe distance would usually be a couple of car lengths. I left about four or five, which was about as much as I could do without losing them. I thanked my lucky stars that it was only 20-odd miles and I hadn't made the mistake of phoning a donkey sanctuary further afield.

Fern called me just as we were getting close to the school gates.

'Are you near?' she said.

'Near enough, we're just by that petrol station,' I said.

I toyed with whether to tell her anything about my morning, but figured it may be best to keep my concerns to myself.

'Are you okay?' she said.

'I'm fine,' I said.

'You seem a little on edge,' said Fern. 'Never work with children or animals, that's what they say, isn't it? Well, don't worry, I'll take care of the kids, if you take care of the animals.'

That was precisely what I was worried about.

The kids were understandably excited. Fern had held off telling them there would be a live donkey onstage until the morning rehearsal. The children had all bounded into school with great big smiles on their faces, swinging carrier bags of costumes in their hands. By the time I pulled into the car park the place was ready to explode.

I'm not sure whose bright idea it was to have us pull into the car park in the middle of lunch break, but that's exactly what happened. It was mayhem. Children were charging about the places like wind-up mice, squeaking and shrieking, laughing and jostling, trading cards, singing songs and throwing tennis balls as hard as they could at the fence. For some reason I thought they'd be so wrapped up in their playground worlds that they wouldn't notice our little convoy be ushered in at the gate, weave our way down the little drive and park up by the emergency exits. But two cars and a horsebox are hardly inconspicuous. It took about four seconds for the children to swarm around us. From all four corners of the playground they huddled so tight I could barely open the door.

I suddenly felt a feeling I was not accustomed to feeling – responsibility. I wound down the window.

'Can we all move away from the cars?' I said. 'I know you all know what's inside, but she gets nervous when there's lots of people around.'

'No, I don't,' joked Polly from her window. 'Oh, do you mean the donkey?'

How was I going to cope with Polly, the donkey and the kids? The word 'donkey' set off the children. They shrieked and giggled and kicked their legs. One child climbed on another's back and rode him round in circles like they were on Blackpool Pleasure Beach.

'I'm sorry, but you're all going to have to get back. Take a big step back, please.'

The kids shuffled back a few millimetres.

'I said a BIG step back!'

They shuffled another few millimetres as if to test me.

Salvation arrived in a familiar form.

'Please! Miss Gilmore!' I bellowed at the top of my lungs. 'How do you make them do what you tell them?'

'Children!' said Miss Gilmore sharply.

A hundred heads swivelled round. One by one they sheepishly slunk away and went back to whatever they'd been doing before the donkey train arrived. Fern walked straight up to me.

'How did you do that?' I said.

'I guess some people have it and some people don't,' said Fern, 'and threatening to make the naughty ones tidy up after the performance today helps.'

Polly opened the door of her Range Rover.

'You must be Polly, we spoke on the phone,' said Fern rushing over. 'Thank you so much for helping us today. It's going to be the thing everyone talks about.'

'For the right reasons, I hope,' Polly said. 'Would you be a sweetie, darling, and fetch my crutches from the back?'

Fern's face froze.

'Your what?' she said.

'My crutches,' said Polly.

Fern turned around and looked at me. I bit my lip and made a sort of apologetic face.

'They're under the outfit,' said Polly.

'The outfit?' I spluttered.

'For the play. Since you said I was going to be onstage I made a little effort for the kids.'

Fern opened the back door of the car to see a costume lying on the seat. She picked up the hanger and lifted out an Abba-esque white boiler suit. Polly had decorated it with sequins and stars.

'Wow,' I said, 'that is…special.'

But that wasn't all. Fern held up a pair of over-sized sunglasses and a halo made out of an old wire coat hanger, wrapped in tinsel.

'What do you think?' said Polly. 'You have to use your imagination.'

'Er…' Fern stumbled around for the words.

'I thought an angel would be the right sort of person to lead the donkey. Or a star, but I figured you'd already have stars, so that could get confusing.'

Polly was officially crackers.

'Genius,' I said, 'that is brilliant.'

'I don't suppose there's any point me wearing it now,' she sighed.

Fern held the halo up in the air and twirled it round.

'That is a shame,' I said, smirking, 'I can just picture it now.'

Fern stopped twirling the halo. She looked at it, then looked at me, then looked at the outfit again.

'What do you think?' she said.

'About what?' I said.

'Come here for a sec,' said Fern to me.

'Oh no,' I said. 'No way.'

'Yes,' said Polly, clapping her hands, 'that's a wonderful idea.'

The roads by the school were lined up and down with cars. You couldn't find a space for half a mile. Eager parents and families had arrived early to get priority seating and lined the front rows, clutching their video cameras. Most of them had been subjected to week after week of rehearsals. The music teacher fancied herself as an *X Factor*-style mentor and the children had put as much rehearsal time into this event as a Lionel Richie stadium tour. The stage was an elaborate set created by the school caretaker and a handful of teaching assistants. They had rigged up a large cardboard cattle shed, which was decorated with anachronistic props they'd borrowed from a local farmer: tractor wheels and grain sacks. There was a line of hay bales over the left-hand portion of the stage to provide seating for the animal chorus line who were busy having their faces painted as the assembly hall filled.

I think nativity plays these days are different from when I was a kid. I don't remember there beings lions and tigers in mine, or reworkings of Take That songs, for that matter. The Angel of the Lord didn't appear to Mary like a Disney fairy godmother, holding a white umbrella above her head and singing Rhianna's smash hit single. In my day, it was pretty much a stony-faced teacher reading a slightly poetic account of a Bible story while we all acted it out and joined in with the Christmas carols.

I waited in Fern's office; I couldn't handle the scrum of the school canteen which had been transformed into a backstage dressing room. It was buzzing with excited and tearful kids, half in and half out of costumes. Fern had given me my script. I flicked through it, looking for the highlighted bits that signalled where I should come in. I didn't have to turn many pages. The donkey appeared quite early on, just after Angel 1 made her visitation accompanied by the R 'n' B Angel chorus. After this, Joseph led Mary to Bethlehem, which was the cue for a ten-year-old boy and me to lead a donkey on which an eight-year-old girl would be balanced, from the right-hand stage to the left. We would walk around the stage a few times and I would then help Mary off the donkey and wait by the edge of the stage. Which was absolutely fine. In fact, it was perfect. For the rest of the performance I could sit out of the limelight, gently patting Rapunzel, hoping nobody I knew was there, and just walk on at the end to give our final bows (that's if donkeys can give bows). I breathed a sigh of relief. This wasn't nearly as bad as I thought. Come to think of it I wondered why I hadn't looked at the script earlier. The school tannoy went. This time not accompanied by birdsong but the sound of an angelic trumpet.

'Please take you seats for the Grand Performance. The show will start in fifteen minutes.'

Not wanting to disrupt the backstage vibe we had decided it was best to introduce Rapunzel and Polly to the kids at the last possible moment. The emergency exit doors in the canteen led straight out into the playground, so we'd draw the curtains and wait outside until our cue. When the head teacher sounded the five-minute tannoy, we'd make our long-awaited appearance.

'Hello, Polly,' I said, 'how's she doing?'

Polly was in the back of the horsebox on her knees. She had a stiff brush looped around her hand and was pulling it through Rapunzel's mane.

'Ooh, Marc,' she said, 'hello. We're just making ourselves look sexy.'

She looked up from the straw that was lining the floor of the box, with a wry wink in her eye. I nodded gingerly.

'Now she's not going to poo everywhere, is she?' I said. 'That would be typical, wouldn't it? The sort of thing that happens on *Blue Peter*.'

'She went about ten minutes ago, I'll show you if you don't believe me,' said Polly reaching for the manure shovel.

'I don't need to see it!' I said. 'I was only asking.'

Polly tipped back her head and laughed.

'You're really enjoying this, aren't you?' I said.

'What?' she said.

Polly reached into her pockets and pulled out a sugar lump. She placed it on the flat of her hand and Rapunzel hoovered it up.

'Will you be ready in five minutes?' I said.

'Oh, we're ready for anything, aren't we, Rapunzel?' said Polly, nuzzling up to her neck. 'We're going to bring the house down.'

At that exact moment Rapunzel turned her head right round, dragged a hoof across the floor of the horsebox and made an almighty snort.

'Whoa,' said Polly, grabbing hold of the reins and holding her head steady. She must have seen the look of panic in my eye.

'She'll be fine,' she said, 'she's an angel. Now go and get yourself ready.'

*

The tannoy sounded for the five-minute call and the children huddled at the side of the stage murmuring and fidgeting, and practising their lines. Thick velvet curtains hung down, and teachers buzzed about like bees, making final adjustments to costumes and trying to keep everyone in groups. The music teacher thanked everybody and wished them all luck.

'Remember everything we learnt in the rehearsals,' she said, 'and you'll be superstars. Just go out there and enjoy yourselves.'

She gave them all a thumbs-up, before slipping out the door and taking her place at the piano. A teaching assistant with a clipboard was playing the role of stage manager. She called everybody to attention.

'We'll be on now in two minutes,' she said, checking her watch, 'I need Mary and Joseph on the stage now, in position. And the angels come to the front and get ready.'

Mary was the sweetest thing you ever saw. She was a little girl called Sophie with bushes of fiery red hair. She had these big green eyes that popped out of her face. As she stood there in a nightdress made out of a bedsheet she looked very, very nervous. Joseph couldn't have been more different. He had buzzed hair, a cheeky grin, and the most infectious laugh. He was wearing a Dennis the Menace dressing gown. Inside out, so there weren't any logos. His mum and gran were in the front row.

'Sophie,' said the stage manager, 'hold on a sec,' and she ran over and tightened the rope belt so the cushion – acting as a baby – wouldn't slip out.

The head teacher was no stranger to theatrics, he was dressed in black tie and tuxedo with a megaphone swinging from his hand. He stepped onto the stage, and the crowd fell silent.

'Lords and ladies, boys and girls,' he bellowed, 'Welcome to the highlight of the school year. There is no need for an introduction so without any further ado, will you turn off your phones, tune in your hearing aids and turn up the applause for the magical story of Mary and Joseph.'

Everyone burst into applause.

The play started well. The music teacher played a few notes on the piano that sounded more like the introduction to *War of the Worlds* than a nativity play and the curtains lifted, revealing two people sleeping in the middle of the stage. So far, so good. A boy shuffled up to the front holding a microphone.

'I am the narrator,' he announced to the room, and he put on a pair of newsreader glasses to give him an air of authority.

'Once upon a time in a land far away there lived a girl called Mary who had a boyfriend called Joseph.'

Joseph sat up and waved. The audience tittered.

'One night when they were asleep, Mary was woken by a rather special visitor.'

At this point the music teacher got up and began to slap the lid of the piano to make a crude drum beat. From the right-hand side of the stage Angel 1 appeared. She was a little girl in her white sheet, and she spun and skipped like a ballerina, twirling above her head a large white umbrella, as she sung a nativitified version of the chorus of Rhianna's smash hit 'Umbrella'. It was a truly eye-opening re-imagination of the celestial appearance to the Virgin. She was joined by the R 'n' B angelic choir for the last bit.

> *When the stars shine, they shine together,*
> *Tell you God is here for ever.*
> *He will always be your friend,*
> *And he'll be there, people, right till the end.*
> *He has sent me with some news,*
> *You are going to have a baby.*
> *And it's going to be a fella,*
> *You can stand under his umbrella.*
> *Ella, ella, ella, eh, eh,*
> *Under his umbrella,*
> *ella, ella, eh, eh.*

The audience broke into peals of applause, whoops and cheers. Angel 1 turned a bright red colour and hugged herself with her arms.

'You must go to Bethlehem because there's an evil man who wants to kill you. Do not fear,' said Angel 1, and she turned and flapped offstage.

Fern grabbed my arm.

'Are you ready?' she whispered to me.

'I think so,' I said, 'I'll go and get Rapunzel.'

Fern was beaming.

'Thank you for this,' she said, and planted a kiss on my cheek.

Polly and Rapunzel were waiting quietly outside the double doors.

'We're on,' I said. 'Let's go.'

Rapunzel stepped over the threshold and we brought her into the rehearsal room. The children went bananas. They had been quietly sitting in little groups, but all that went out the window as some charged forward to stroke her and others ran for cover and hid behind the tables.

'Don't crowd her,' I said. 'She's very shy.'

I turned to look at Polly. She looked like she was in heaven.

'She's called Rapunzel,' she said, and produced some sugar lumps from her pocket.

'Everyone back to where you were,' said Fern. 'Marc, I think it's your cue.'

Back onstage, Mary had just been explaining the angel's visit to Joseph and now Joseph was taking control.

'Let's go to Bethlehem,' he said, 'where is my trusty steed?'

The stage manager beckoned me.

'You're on,' she said.

There are some moments in life that make you sit back and think about who you are, what you're about, and what on earth you're doing. This was certainly one of those. Five years of vet school and my past few years of professional work had all been building up to the day that I dressed in a white lady's boiler suit adorned with sequins and sparkles and a coat hanger crown wrapped in tinsel and walked onto the stage of a primary school, leading a rescue donkey upon which was sitting an eight-year-old girl.

I took a deep breath and stepped onto that stage. At first all the audience could see was a grown man in a sequinned boiler suit and there was an audible murmur of surprise. I gave Rapunzel a little tug, and expected her to join me. But Rapunzel wouldn't move. I looked behind me. She just stood there, staring.

'Come on, girl,' I said, 'this is your moment.'

I gave her another little tug. I looked out at a sea of bemused faces.

'Come on, slowcoach,' said Joseph, ad-libbing.

'All right,' I said, 'hold your horses.'

The audience laughed.

With another tug Rapunzel picked up her hooves and finally ventured out onstage. Little kids jumped onto their chairs. Adults zoomed in their video cameras. Everyone shrieked and squealed. My heart was pounding. *It'll all be over in a few minutes*, I kept telling myself,

A little girl walked to the front of the stage and, accompanied by the music teacher on the piano, she sung the first verse of 'Little Donkey'. This was to be the soundtrack to the great donkey ride to Bethlehem. I helped Mary onto the back of the donkey and she clung on for dear life as we very slowly walked three laps of the stage. Camera bulbs flashed, people cheered, this was what everyone would talk about. I looked down at my ridiculous outfit as we plodded round the stage again. Luckily my name wasn't in the programme, so any photos from this event wouldn't be tagged on Facebook. But then as we turned the corner I caught sight of a face I recognised in the second row. Oh God. Surely it couldn't be? Could it? The audience was behind me now so I couldn't turn around to check. We walked the length of the back of the stage and turned around for the final time. I was now looking straight to where she was sitting. She was standing up and cheering, and then all of a sudden I recognised the person sitting next to her. This small round

Welsh lady put her fingers in her mouth and blew a wolf-whistle.

'Go Marc!' she yelled. 'Whooo-yeah!'

Ruth and Gloria.

What were they doing here?

'We love you, Marc!' shouted Ruth.

Oh God! Please tell me they don't have a camera.

As I lifted Mary down from the back of the donkey and turned to the audience for the final time, Ruth was snapping away frantically. This was the end of the world. Well, it wasn't, quite, yet.

I sat offstage, quietly fuming to myself. How did I end up in a white sequinned boiler suit on stage in front of millions (almost) of people? I picked at the stupid pieces of glitter and sulked. How dare Ruth and Gloria come and ruin my moment? I couldn't bring myself to poke my head around the curtains but I imagined them clutching their stomachs from laughing so hard and fishing tissues out of their handbags to wipe away the tears. Rapunzel stood there patiently and watched as Mary and Joseph were turned away by a serious of underage innkeepers with decidedly suspect beards.

'What are we going to do?' said Joseph.

'You can sleep in the cattle shed,' said the innkeeper.

The narrator appeared again in his newsreader specs.

'That night, when everyone was sleeping,' he said, 'Mary and Joseph had a special delivery...'

A boy dressed as a stork flapped in from the side of the stage with a plastic doll in a pillowcase.

'… it was a baby boy and they named him Jesus.'

The audience was lapping it up.

I sunk my hands in my pockets. My fingers landed on something hard and lumpy, wrapped in rustly paper. At the sound of it Rapunzel's head shot round. Sugar lumps. Of course.

'You can't have them now,' I whispered.

She made eyes at me.

'At the end,' I said, 'there's a good girl.'

The paper rustled again as I carefully withdrew my hand from my pocket. A flicker flashed across Rapunzel's face and without a second thought she went for it. She pulled her head in and wrapped her teeth around the pocket of my boiler suit.

'No!' I said trying to shoe her away. 'Rapunzel, stop!'

Her teeth were strong. She tugged. I heard the pocket tear.

'Rapunzel!'

I was raising my voice now. With that she tugged her head and heaved the rope out of my hands. The children on the stage stopped and stared.

'Oh God!' I said. 'Rapunzel!'

Then she bolted. Rapunzel was off like a rocket. She tore across the stage, making a beeline for the crib. The children dived this way and that, Joseph hid under a blanket and Mary scrambled behind a hay bale. Rapunzel seized Baby Jesus by his babygro, and whipped him over her head. She turned to face the audience in the middle of the stage, frozen like a rabbit in the headlights. The whole place rose to its feet. Mary burst into tears.

'It's okay, it's okay,' I said, as much for my benefit as everyone else's. I bent down and tried to grab the rope, but every time I reached for it the donkey whipped her head round and sent the rope flying. The head teacher ditched his megaphone and tried to clear the front two rows. Ruth and Gloria ran to the stage and asked if I needed help. Rapunzel just stood there, staring out as if she knew all the cameras were trained at her, and drank up all the attention.

It took ten minutes after we caught the donkey before the kids were able to go back onstage. The animal chorus was in tears, and Mary was a jitter of nerves. The performance was a success in some respects: we raised eight hundred pounds for the sanctuary and most of the parents in the audience got a far more entertaining show than they could possibly have expected, and nobody got hurt. It took four of us to pen Rapunzel into a corner of the assembly hall. I eventually got hold of the rope and led her back to the horsebox. I made my exit as soon as I could.

*

I returned to the practice in the evening to find that the footage of the fiasco had already been widely circulated. George had taken the liberty of replacing my photo on the 'Meet the Team' board with a picture of Donkey from Shrek.

Merry Christmas everyone.

What else is there to say?

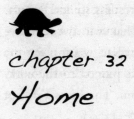

chapter 32
Home

I worked through the Christmas weekend, waiting by the phone for emergency calls, while families up and down the country played charades, yelled at each other and slept off the turkey. We had sorted out a rota. Ruth had the weekend off to spend with her family, and then I was with mine for next couple of days, so the practice was always covered, but it meant it was just me on Christmas Day, watching the movies and the Christmas specials, eating a takeaway pizza (turkey, naturally) with my feet up on the practice sofa, thinking about things. There were no spoons stirring herbal teas, no joking or dancing to MTV. It was quiet, eerie and reflective. But then that time between Christmas and New Year is made for that sort of thing. Routines stop and you step out of real life for a little bit. Most often this takes place at home with other people around, people who know you the best, your family. There isn't that much to do, apart from eat, drink, catch up, play games and think about life, and what you're doing, and everywhere you look there are reminders of the person you once were: the wide-eyed

boy, the awkward teenager, the restless student return-
ing in the holidays. But for me that year, the reflective
time started in the office. The silent waiting for the
phone to ring. The knick-knacks pinned to the corkboard. The Indian takeaway menu. The cards I'd kept
above my desk. I'd built that place, I did it.

I woke up on Boxing Day morning still in the same
place on the practice couch. My overnight bag was on
the chair. I brushed my teeth in the bathroom mirror,
and stared at the man looking back at me. As I drove out
of the car park I turned over the events of the year in my
head. I walked back in my mind into the meeting room
of my old practice and saw the old partners gathered in
a ring telling me I was too immature, that no one wanted
to work with me, and I didn't know the first thing about
business. I thought back to the frustrating phone call
with my parents when Mum put the phone down and
Dad told me I needed to 'settle down'. I thought about
the first day with the new partners, about meeting Ruth
with her weird teas and cleanses, and Gloria with her
warm Welsh ways, about the biker with the budgie,
Chickens the rattling Labrador, Mrs Lopez and the cat
who laid the egg. I thought about Fleur and her gerbils,
the Siamese twins, Lord Horncastle, Dan and Fern. It
had been nothing if not a roller coaster ride.

The passenger seat was covered with gifts, you could
barely see the fabric: a large box from Ruth, a bottle of

something from Gloria, a cute little gift from Fern, wrapped in ivy green paper and tied with a large shiny bow. I hadn't known them a year before but they were like family now. Before I got on my way back to the place I used to call home there was still one small visit to make. I swore I'd never appear in a nativity play again, but I could still be Father Christmas.

It was a short drive. I pulled up outside the house and reached into the glove compartment. I pulled out a present I'd wrapped up the night before in shiny red paper. I'm dreadful at gift-wrapping so the whole thing was done up in metres of tape. I sat in my seat and looked at the house. The lights were on, the place looked warm. There was a Christmas tree in the window with dancing lights, and two sets of wellington boots standing patiently by the front door. It was a perfect picture of Christmas. I stood outside the door and rung the bell. There were noises from inside, footsteps getting louder, then Julie, Donny's mother, opened the door. She was wearing an apron and oven gloves, and did a double take.

'Marc! Hello, Marc. What a surprise! Happy Christmas.' She gave me a hug and said, 'What are you doing here?'

'Just dropping something off,' I said. 'I got a little gift for Donny.'

Julie's eyes went wide. 'For Donny?' she said.

'It's just a little thing,' I said, 'but when you talked about him…well, anyway, I thought he'd like it.'

I handed over the gift, a war game for Donny's computer.

'Happy Christmas from me and Holly the fox.'

Dad was pleased. I got to London in record time, and was not only there before lunch was served, but I made it in time for beer and peanuts. My parents aren't big drinkers, but they always like to put beer in the fridge for when I come home.

'We got you some Boddingtons,' said Mum, with that look on her face that said 'aren't you impressed I remembered?'. 'That *is* the one you really like isn't it?' she said.

Mum must have seen me order it once in a pub. She'd been supplying me with Boddingtons for years. I hadn't the heart to tell her that I don't really have a favourite, and if I did, it wouldn't be Boddingtons. More likely Doom Bar.

'Perfect,' I said.

Mum came over and gave me another hug.

'It's so good to have you back,' she said. 'Lunch will be a few minutes. Your father's in the lounge, watching something about penguins.'

'It's *Happy Feet*!' called Dad.

Mum is the multiple-hug, fuss-about, good-to-see-you type, Dad's way of showing how excited he is to see you was to sit in his chair and not move a muscle.

'When do you want to do presents?' said Mum. 'Your father and I have done ours already.'

She turned left and right to show off her earrings.

'Amazing!' I said. 'They look lovely.'

I was still in my coat and holding my bags.

'Let the boy sit down,' Dad said.

'I know, but I'm excited,' said Mum.

'But he's only just got in,' Dad pointed out.

'I know, but I can't help it,' she replied. She grabbed my arm. 'I'm sorry, darling, I'm not fussing you, am I?'

I sat in the lounge and shovelled handfuls of peanuts into my mouth while cartoon penguins danced about the television screen.

'How's work?' Dad said, after a minute or two.

'Good,' I said, 'we're doing well. We may have to expand.'

Dad said nothing.

We watched the television in silence for a bit.

'I always knew you could do it, son,' he said proudly. 'It's in the Abraham genes.'

I smiled.

Mum insisted on watching me open my presents. This year's haul went something like this: Ruth gave me a karaoke machine with a little note which said – *for office use only*, Gloria had hilariously wrapped up a bottle of Lambrini, and Fern's gift, was, well, an Adopt-a-Donkey

Gift pack – according to the certificate I was now the proud sponsor of a handsome donkey called Jazzy.

'You've not opened this one,' said Mum.

She whipped out a present from behind her back, grinning from ear to ear.

'You can take it back if you don't like it,' she said.

She always said this.

'Thanks,' I said, and paused. 'Shall I open it now?'

'Go on,' she said. 'Tony, he's opening our present.'

Dad craned in to watch. 'What is it?' he said.

I tore a small corner of paper and slowly unpeeled the wrapping. Underneath was a plain white box. I looked at Mum. She smiled back.

'Open the top,' she said.

I tucked my fingernails in, and carefully opened the lid. Inside was a large white globe.

'Ah,' I said, 'thanks, Mum.'

I had no idea what it was.

And then I saw the instruction manual – 'How to Operate Your Seasonal Affective Disorder Lamp'. I looked at my mother. She was glowing.

'For your condition,' she said, and she gave me hug.

I rested my chin on her shoulder and looked up at a school photo propped on the piano.

'Thanks, Mum,' I said, 'it's good to be home.'

Acknowledgements

My first shout-out goes to Davey without whose help this book would not have been possible. A massive thanks also to both Charlotte and Liz at Ebury Press for their patience and guidance through the whole writing process. And thanks to Kate and Ivan for setting the wheels in motion and bringing the whole team together in the first place.

My amazing night nurse Ruth! We've shared some of the most incredible and surreal moments on our hundreds of nights on call together; singing 'Purple Rain' at 5am at the tops of our voices whilst mopping the operating theatre floor stands out. Thanks also to lovely receptionist Gloria, and to Lynda, Nicky, Shirley, Niki and Sally – all absolutely brilliant nurses.

Mum, Dad, Danielle, Nathan and Jordan, the late Oma and Opi, and Grandma Dudu – a survivor of the Holocaust and the bravest, most inspiring positive-thinking person I know.

Local vet Tony Lewis who I volunteered with Saturday mornings and school holidays who taught me about customer service and the importance of always putting the animal's welfare first.

To the great Victoria Stilwell and Paul O'Grady for believing in me and their invaluable input in turning me into a fully-fledged TV vet with the platform to help educate millions of pet owners. And of course to my lovely agent Debs who always knows best!

To best mate 'Doom Brother' Russ, as well as Pacey, Ged, Dave, Nads, Tanya, Kim, Tine, Mark, Andy, Nigel and Sam for all their laughs and incredible unrelenting support – much appreciated guys.

And finally to my beloved hometown Brighton with its unique sunsets and seascapes; one can never fail to be inspired here.